C^{THE}...

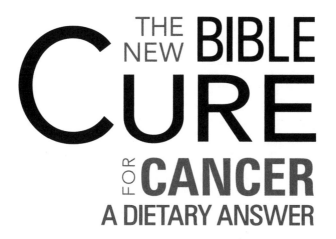

THE NEW BIBLE

CURE

FOR **CANCER**

A DIETARY ANSWER

DON COLBERT, MD

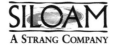

SILOAM

A STRANG COMPANY

Most Strang Communications Book Group products are available at special quantity discounts for bulk purchase for sales promotions, premiums, fund-raising, and educational needs. For details, write Strang Communications Book Group, 600 Rinehart Road, Lake Mary, Florida 32746, or telephone (407) 333-0600.

THE NEW BIBLE CURE FOR CANCER by Don Colbert, MD
Published by Siloam
A Strang Company
600 Rinehart Road
Lake Mary, Florida 32746
www.strangbookgroup.com

Unless otherwise stated, Scripture quotations are from the Holy Bible, New Living Translation, copyright © 1996, 2004. Used by permission of Tyndale House Publishers, Inc., Wheaton, IL 60189. All rights reserved.

Scripture quotations marked NKJV are from the New King James Version of the Bible. Copyright © 1979, 1980, 1982 by Thomas Nelson, Inc., publishers. Used by permission.

Library of Congress Cataloging-in-Publication Data
Colbert, Don.
  The new Bible cure for cancer / Don Colbert. -- [Rev. and updated].
       p. cm.
  Rev. ed. of: The Bible cure for cancer.
  Includes bibliographical references.
  ISBN 978-1-59979-866-0

1. Cancer. 2. Cancer--Alternative treatment. 3. Cancer--Religious aspects--Christianity. I. Colbert, Don. Bible cure for cancer. II. Title.

RC254.C65 2010

616.99'4--dc22

2010023366

10 11 12 13 — 9 8 7 6 5 4 3 2 1

Printed in the United States of America

CONTENTS

A NEW BIBLE CURE WITH NEW HOPE FOR CANCER

F IRST, THE BAD news: cancer is the second leading cause of death in the United States behind cardiovascular disease, killing more than half a million people every year. There are also about 1.5 million new cases each year. Cancer causes nearly one in every four deaths. Men face a slightly less than one-in-two lifetime risk of developing cancer, while women face a little more than a one-in-three chance. If you smoke, you are twenty-three times more likely to develop cancer than if you do not. Because of these odds, it is very likely that you or someone you love will face cancer sometime in your lifetime. Cancer costs America over $228 billion a year.[1]

What could be good news after all that? Very simply this: *cancer is beatable* and *preventable*. In fact, cancer is on the decline, and those who have survived cancer are living longer and healthier than ever before.[2]

More than two-thirds of the causes of cancer are things within our day-to-day control.[3] There are also foods and nutrients we can add to our daily routine to reduce our risks even further. Cancer may be a Goliath of a problem in the United States today, but you have the same God on your side who helped the Goliath-killer. If you ask Him and heed His wisdom, you can beat the giant of cancer as well.

Your first victory over cancer must be on the battlefield of fear. Most people want to put their heads in the sand and ignore this kind of a problem, but just by picking up this book, you have shown you are different. I encourage you to make a bold decision to stand up against this giant and reach beyond fear to discover the hope and faith possible through *The New Bible Cure for Cancer*.

The path to victory is clearer and better plotted out today than ever before. Modern medicine, along with cutting-edge nutritional therapies—all built upon good nutrition and sound principles of daily living—make the threat of cancer much less lethal than it once was. Add to this a bold Christian faith to lay hold of the promises of God in Scripture for your health, and you have all you need to arm you against this fearful Goliath and equip you to face any physical or spiritual onslaught. After all, the Word of God says:

> Let all that I am praise the LORD; may I never forget the good things he does for me. He forgives all my sins and heals all my diseases.
>
> —PSALM 103:2–3

I have personally witnessed many people who have fought this battle against cancer and triumphed. This war is winnable, and many have already won it. However, an ounce of prevention is worth a pound of cure, and sound nutritional dietary and lifestyle principles prevent cancer.

The battle must begin today, however. Every day, your immune system needs to be ready to detect and destroy cancer cells before they obtain a foothold. Around you and within you are a myriad of cancer-causing agents that come through the air you breathe, the food you eat, and the beverages you drink. The information in this book will show you what to do to arm your immune system, focusing especially upon how nutrition can be a key player in this fight. God has provided both natural and supernatural agents to battle cancer and help you win the war. Because of all this, you have nothing to fear. After all, "God has not given us a spirit of fear, but of power and of love and of a sound mind" (2 Tim. 1:7, NKJV).

Welcome to yet another hope-filled book in the Bible Cure series to help you know how to keep the temple of your body fit and healthy. In this series of books, you will uncover God's divine plan of health for body, soul, and spirit through modern medicine, good nutrition, and the medicinal power of Scripture and prayer.

Originally published as *The Bible Cure for Cancer* in 1999, *The New Bible Cure for Cancer* has been revised and updated with the latest medical research on this disease. If you compare it side by side with the previous edition, you'll see that it's also larger, allowing me to expand greatly upon the information provided in the previous edition and provide you with a deeper understanding of what you face and how to overcome it.

Unchanged from the previous edition are the timeless, life-changing, and healing scriptures throughout this book that will strengthen and encourage your spirit and soul. The proven principles, truths, and guidelines in these passages anchor the practical and medical insights also contained in this book. They will effectively focus your prayers, thoughts, and actions so you can step into God's plan of divine health for you—a plan that includes victory over cancer.

Another change since the original *The Bible Cure for Cancer* was published is that I've released a very important book *The Seven Pillars of Health.* I encourage you to read it, because the principles of health it contains are the foundation to healthy living that will affect all areas of your life. It sets the stage for everything you will ever read in any other book I've published—including this one.

I pray that these spiritual and practical suggestions for health, nutrition, and fitness will bring wholeness to your life, increase your spiritual understanding, and strengthen your ability to worship and serve God.

—DON COLBERT, MD

A **BIBLE CURE** Prayer for You

Jesus, I thank You that You died on the cross to deliver me from fear and to overcome the power of sickness and death. I thank You that Your name is above every name, and the power of cancer is broken in my life and the lives of my loved ones. Lord Jesus, touch my body at this moment with Your healing power. Cleanse my mind from fear and my body from disease. Give me wisdom to live a healthy life that brings honor to You for the wonderful Creator that You are. In the mighty name of Jesus Christ, according to the Word of God, I declare that in Christ I have victory over cancer. The power of this disease is broken in my life and in the lives of those I love. Amen.

Chapter 1

SQUELCHING THE CELL REBELLION

LEANOR ROOSEVELT SAID, "I gain strength, courage, and confidence by every experience in which I must stop and look fear in the face."[1] This is exactly what we need to do with the face of cancer. While cancer has been a Goliath of a killer in recent decades, it is on the decline because more and more people are learning that it is beatable and are changing their habits accordingly. God's wisdom on how we should live and what we should eat is at the foundation of all who are preventing and beating cancer today through better nutrition, wholesome living, and overcoming faith. Understanding this wisdom is more important today then ever.

In addition to the powerful breakthroughs experienced in the medical arena, miracles by the healing touch of God happen every day. Instantaneous miracles are performed in a moment by the power of the Holy Spirit. I have seen many people whose triumph over cancer, even in its advanced stages, can only be described as miraculous. And I know other medical doctors who would agree that they too have witnessed such dramatic occurrences. However, generally God *won't* do what you *can* do. You must change your diet and lifestyle to prevent cancer.

I have also witnessed numerous other healings that took place over a longer period of time. These patients pray, trust God's Word, and use natural therapies that include a healthy diet, good nutrition, supplements, detoxification measures, and lifestyle changes. This approach provides an arsenal of weapons to battle the many factors that cause cancer.

> Who Himself bore our sins in His own body on the tree, that we, having died to sins, might live for righteousness—by whose stripes you were healed.
> —1 PETER 2:24, NKJV

GOD'S DESIGN FOR PERSONAL HEALTH CARE

In order to understand how the Bible cure defeats cancer, it is important to first know how cancer develops. We actually use the word *cancer* to describe a vast and varied number of processes that are so complex and widespread that science is still working around the clock to try to understand and name them all. Researchers are far from completely understanding all of the elements that can cause cancer as well as all the different abnormal processes in the body that allow it to grow and spread. However, with that said, all of them do seem to follow a similar general pattern, and by doing what we can to prevent that pattern, we can also prevent cancer from forming, keep it from spreading, or sometimes even cause it to self-destruct.

Perhaps the best analogy for understanding how cancer forms is to think of your body as a nation made up of different cities and towns that all have functions that contribute to the health of the overall whole. Each of these cities has to work together and communicate with each other through various systems, like the cardiovascular, lymphatic, and nervous systems, which act as highways to transport nutrients, send signals, or carry away waste. Each city is made up of millions of cells that each perform a unique function. All your "cities" together are home to approximately 60 trillion cells. The body is producing new cells all of the time as it needs one thing or another; each cell then performs its task and eventually dies after a certain period of time so that the body can maintain balances of what it needs and what it doesn't need. These dead cells are then cleared away and replaced by new cells. In fact, your body replaces approximately 90 to 95 percent of its mass on a cellular level every two years or so through the healthy creation, function, death, and then clearing away of your cells.

Cells are manufactured according to the genetic code embedded in each, and for the most part after their own kind—in other words, intestinal cells produce other intestinal cells, endothelial cells (those that make up the inside wall of your blood vessels) produce other endothelial cells, liver cells produce other liver cells, and so on. Of course, with so many billions of new cells being made all of the time, every once in a while there is a mistake—a "typo" in the copying of the correct parts of the genetic code into the production of a new cell. This can simply be a mistake, or it can be caused by any number of *carcinogens*, including free radicals, foreign contaminants, or radiation, just to name a few. The truth of the matter is that these typos happen rather frequently, and while they are potentially the first stage of cancer, most of the time they do not become cancer because they are handled by the "police force" of your immune system without incident.

The immune system is both the smallest and the largest system of the body. It has no organs or pathways of its own and is made up of numerous cells, including lymphocytes (white blood cells), phagocytes, natural killer (NK) cells, and other components, including antibodies, complement, and interferons. These immune cells travel throughout every other system of the body as tiny "police officers" looking for invaders or rebels to capture and expel. The immune cells know how to identify cells and substances in the body that are either friendly and native (normal cells, proteins, enzymes, etc.) or unfriendly and foreign (bacteria, viruses, dead cells, "typos," antigens, etc.). When the immune cells find these, figuratively speaking they grab hold of them, neutralize them, and then escort them to the nearest exit as best they can. The foot soldiers of the immune system are the lymphocytes, of which there are two types: T lymphocytes, which are from the thymus gland, and B lymphocytes (B cells), which are from the bone marrow.

Of these tiny "agents of order" within the body, the NK cells are the most potent anticancer fighters. While most immune system lymphocytes are specially designed to fight a specific "invader" (which is how immunity to a new disease is formed), NK cells can attack and destroy rebel cells they have never seen before. This gives them much better range and efficiency than the lymphocytes and phagocytes. Understanding what to do to keep these cells at healthy levels and peak performance is one of the best things we can do to prevent and fight cancer.

When the immune system is working efficiently, we are healthy and thriving, but when it becomes weakened or overwhelmed, we may get "sick" in various ways. When this happens over a long period of time, we open the door for cancer to form and spread in our bodies.

How Typos Become Cancer

So you see that just because the body produces typos—which are more scientifically referred to as *mutations*—it doesn't mean you have cancer. In fact, your body typically produces numerous mutations each day without a problem because your immune system is on top of things. These mutated cells are not cancerous in and of themselves and, as a rule, are easily handled by the immune system. These mutated cells, however, are useless workers in the body, ill equipped to perform the function for which they were created or, for that matter, any other function useful to the body.

Trouble begins when these useless cells begin reproducing themselves, making duplicate copies of their own mistaken identities. This process is referred to as the *initiation* of cancer. *Initiated* cells cannot be repaired or reversed; they can only be destroyed and removed. *Initiation* is similar to the spreading of rebellion or mutiny, as specific cells no longer perform the function for which they were designed but simply reproduce other rebellious cells. They also show no allegiance to the normal commands of the body, replicating without being told to do so. Yet initiated cells are still not cancer cells.

However, initiated cells can become cancer when they meet a *promoter*. *Promoters* are carcinogenic substances, including certain hormones, that encourage initiated cells to start reproducing rapidly and sometimes uncontrollably. Promoters have no effect on normal cells, and usually the promotion process can be reversed; thus, it is possible to dissolve tumors, but promotion is the first step where mutated cells are actually considered cancerous.

In the third stage the mutated cells go through is the *progression stage*. In this stage the mutated and transformed cell gains its independence and becomes malignant and invasive. It begins to invade the surrounding tissues and is capable of infinite reproduction. It is resistant to apoptosis, or cellular suicide. It forms new blood vessels and metastasizes. These cancerous tumors begin to form new blood vessels to both feed itself and invade and spread throughout the body, bent on the destruction and disruption of normal processes—completely devastating to everything they encounter. Not only do these tumors now compete with normal cells for food, but they also further weaken "business as usual" in the body. To make it worse, these cells never fully mature, staying in a perpetual adolescent rebellion. Eventually, if they are not stopped, they will damage and destroy everything that they encounter to the point of killing the very body that feeds them.

This is a long, involved process that takes years and requires the breakdown of several defensive systems for the cancer to grow and flourish. This is why the likelihood of cancer increases with age. There are many other factors that take a toll on our bodies—for example, smoking; poor nutrition; lack of sleep; low natural killer cell counts; genetic susceptibilities; exposure to pollution, radiation, contaminants, and toxins; excessive stress, trauma; obesity; lack of exercise; low levels of oxygen in our bodies; alcohol abuse; or any number of other contributing factors. In fact, there are at least five different things that must happen in order for cancer to thrive and grow.

A **BIBLE CURE** *Health Fact*

The Five Essentials for Cancer Growth

1. Initiated cells replicate without chemical signals from the body instructing them to do so.
2. Initiated cells ignore orders to stop growing or die (*apoptosis*, programmed cell death), given from nearby cells that perceive them as a threat.
3. The tumor that is forming "outsmarts" the immune system in some way so that the immune system fails in identifying, attacking, or killing or cancer cells, thus allowing the tumor to live on and reproduce without interruption.
4. The tumor "hijacks" blood flow—often forming new blood vessel pathways in a process called *angiogenesis*—in order to obtain the nutrients it needs to grow.
5. The tumor grows large enough that it begins to break off parts of itself to spread (a process called *metastasis*) and begins new cancerous colonies throughout the body in various different organs and systems.

CONTROLLING THE TIPPING POINT

For all of these to happen, something has to "tip the scale" in the wrong direction. The good news about that is it means the scale can also be tipped in the right direction, and, oddly enough, there are not that many different things that you have to do to start "tipping" the advantage against cancer back in your favor.

In fact, roughly two-thirds of cancer risks can be reduced by addressing two areas: (1) stopping smoking and/or avoiding secondhand smoke, and (2) eating a proper, nutritious diet. There are more than 4,000 chemicals in cigarette smoke; at least 250 are known to be harmful, and more than 50 have been found to cause cancer.[2] You will reduce your risk of contracting cancer by roughly 30 percent by stopping smoking, and roughly another third can be controlled by eating properly and getting the proper nutrients and supplements. You can add an additional 5 percent decrease in cancer risk if you throw in exercise and maintain a healthy weight.[3] Thus, if you don't smoke and aren't around smokers, the most important thing you can do is follow this Bible cure to adjust your diet, take specific nutrients and supplements, exercise regularly, and maintain a healthy weight for your height.

Of the remaining roughly one-third of risks factors, about half of those (15 percent) have to do with hereditary or genetic factors. Approximately 5 percent are due to infections such as HPV (human papillomavirus) causing cervical cancer, and about 5 percent are from toxic exposure. For example:

- The Environmental Protection Agency (EPA) has classified benzene as a Class A carcinogen due to its link to an increased risk of leukemia. It is used in many of the products we encounter every day—carpet cleaners, cleaning fluids, conditioners, detergents, dyes, enamel sprays, furniture, gasoline, nail polishes, paint, paint removers, paint thinners, plastics, solvents, spot removers, spray acrylics, spray paints, stains/lacquers, vinyl floorings, wood finishes, wood lighteners, wood preservatives, and many other man-made products.[4]

- Perchloroethylene (also called perc, PCE, and tetrachloroethylene) and 1-1-1 trichloroethane solvents, found in spot removers and carpet cleaners, can cause liver and kidney damage if ingested. Perc, determined to be a carcinogen by the Department of Health and Human Services, has caused liver and kidney tumors in laboratory animals.[5] Perc is commonly used in dry cleaning.

- Chlorine is added to public drinking water as a public health measure to kill microorganisms. But chlorine is not entirely safe. It can combine with organic materials to form *trihalomethanes*— a cancer-promoting substance. Bladder cancer has been linked to chlorinated drinking water in ten out of the eleven most reliable studies.

The remaining small percentage is comprised of exposure to alcohol, drugs, UV exposure, pollution, or a handful of other factors too small in percentage and too numerous to list here.[6]

Remarkably, the Bible has answers for the vast majority of these risk factors. For example, the ancient Hebrew texts of the Bible reveal guidelines for eating that can lower your cancer risk. One such thing is the directive to avoid animal fats. As the Bible declares:

You must never eat any fat or blood. This is a perma-
nent law for you, and it must be observed from
generation to generation, wherever you live.

—LEVITICUS 3:17

The fat referred to in this passage comes from the visceral fat
surrounding organs or the portions of meat containing the most
dangerous substances: not only does this fat contain toxins,
pesticides, and other chemicals, but it also contains low-density
lipoproteins, or what is commonly referred to as LDL cholesterol.
As you'll see in the following chapters, Scripture also suggests
that natural fruits and vegetables provide the best nutrition for
our bodies. Problems in the average westerner's diet occur when
daily meals ignore biblical guidelines and consist of:

- Excessive intake of meats

- Excessive animal fat and other fats, including
  inflammatory and toxic oils, trans fats, and fried
  foods

- Excessive sugar and high-glycemic foods (such as
  white flour), which weaken the immune system

- Devitalized foods, including salt, processed
  foods, junk food, and many fast foods

- Toxins in our food, such as nitrites and nitrates
  in processed foods and smoked and cured meats

- Heavy metals, including mercury (found in many fish and silver fillings), as well as other toxic metals and chemicals

Thankfully, God has provided for us both natural methods and supernatural power to overcome any and all risks for letting cancer develop unchecked within us. So don't quit. Don't give up. Don't surrender to fear. Cancer is not the last word—God's Word is!

Always remember that you aren't helpless against cancer. You can begin now to take some practical, positive steps toward defeating it. Just start implementing my suggested "prescriptions" in each chapter. (However, since I cannot give you all the answers for your unique situation, always consult a physician as well to determine the prevention or treatment plan that's best for you.)

The great gospel singer Pearl Bailey once said, "People see God every day; they just don't recognize Him."[7] In your battle with cancer, look for God in everything around you. Recognize His presence in all you do, for He cares for you with a love that runs deeper than the oceans.

> God is our refuge and strength, always ready to help in times of trouble. So we will not fear when earthquakes come and the mountains crumble into the sea.
> —PSALM 46:1–2

A **BIBLE CURE** Prayer for You

Father, in the name of Jesus, I ask that Your healing power fill my body and that the presence of the Holy Spirit would trip up the cancer-causing cycle within me. I ask that Your Holy Spirit invigorate my immune system, which You designed to keep me healthy, and guide it to wipe out all the mutated cells.

As You do, I pledge to add the wisdom of Your Bible cure to my faith and actions and be ruled by Your Word on what I was designed to eat and not be ruled by my fleshly appetites. Help me overcome my cravings as I seek to get to and maintain a healthy weight, that I would have more energy and greater alertness to build Your kingdom upon this earth.

I thank You in the name above every name, Jesus Christ, the great Healer. Amen.

A **BIBLE CURE** *Prescription*

Take Some First Steps

Ready to take some first steps in fighting cancer? Here's a summary list of some practical things you can start doing right now. Check the ones you'd like to begin today:

❑ I'll limit my intake of red meat to 18 ounces or less a week and choose leaner cuts.

❑ I'll begin reevaluating my diet and thinking about healthier eating habits.

❑ I'll limit my high-fat foods, especially fried foods and high-fat meats. I'll avoid trans fats.

❑ I'll avoid cigarette smoke, and I will determine never to smoke or to quit if I do smoke. I'll avoid secondhand smoke.

❑ I'll take time to read and memorize God's Word, especially scriptural promises for healing.

❑ I'll determine to choose faith and reject fear, because the Bible says Jesus Christ defeated cancer and disease.

Chapter 2

THE CANCER-DEFEATING DIET PLAN

W<small>E ARE ALL</small> creatures of habits that have been formed by the cultures we live in. We like to eat certain things because that is simply the way we were raised by our parents. It is part of who we are and where we live in the world. I was raised on southern cooking in Mississippi, where they fried almost everything, put bacon grease in the vegetables, smothered biscuits with gravy, and drank sweet tea.

> Then God said, "Look! I have given you every seed-bearing plant throughout the earth and all the fruit trees for your food."
>
> —G<small>ENESIS</small> 1:29

When we eat the kind of diet the Creator of our bodies intended, we naturally build a strong immune system that defends against cancer as well as other diseases. In fact, it has been found that the very same diet that Jesus probably ate—one based on the eating habits in Israel and other Mediterranean countries and one that includes a good deal of fruits and vegetables—is the healthiest in the world.

THE MEDITERRANEAN DIET

According to a recent study, "People who eat a Mediterranean-style diet rich in fruits, vegetables, whole grains, olive oil, and fish have at least a 25 percent reduced risk of dying from heart disease and cancer."[1] This is because the Mediterranean diet derives roughly 30 to 40 percent of its calories from healthy fats (coming from things like olive oil, avocados, nuts, and fish) and about 40 to 50 percent from healthy carbohydrates like fruits, vegetables, and whole grains. Researchers also surmised that it was not any one component of this diet that makes it preventative, but the overall combination of foods, as well as avoiding foods that are potentially harmful, such as excessive calories from omega-6 oils, butter, sweets, and meats. Combined with daily exercise, this is a powerful diet for living a longer and healthier life. Another study estimated that up to 25 percent of the incidence of colorectal cancer, about 15 percent of the incidence of breast cancer, and about 10 percent of the incidence of prostate cancer could be prevented if we shifted from a common Western diet to a traditional Mediterranean one.[2]

The Mediterranean diet is made up primarily of the foods listed below. (For a more detailed look at the Mediterranean diet, refer to my books *Dr. Colbert's "I Can Do This" Diet*, *Eat This and Live!* and *What Would Jesus Eat?*)

- *Extra-virgin olive oil*—replaces most fats, oils, butter, and margarine. It is used in salads as well as for cooking. Extra-virgin olive oil strengthens the immune system.

- *Bread*—consumed daily and is prepared as whole-grain, dark, chewy, crusty loaves. Eat whole-grain breads and sprouted breads such as Ezekiel 4:9 bread, and avoid white processed bread.

- *Thick, whole-grain pasta; brown or wild rice; couscous; bulgur; potatoes*—often served with fresh vegetables and herbs, sautéed in olive oil, and occasionally served with small quantities of lean beef

- *Fruit*—preferably raw, two to three pieces daily

- *Nuts*—especially pecans and almonds; at least ten per day

- *Beans*—including pintos, great northern, navy, and kidney beans. Beans and lentil soups are very popular (prepared with a small amount of extra-virgin olive oil). Have at least ½ cup of beans, three to four times weekly.

- *Vegetables*—dark green variety, especially in salads. Eat at least one serving of the following daily: cabbage, broccoli, cauliflower, turnip greens, mustard greens, carrots, spinach, or sweet potatoes—raw or steamed as briefly as possible.

- *Small amounts of low-fat organic cheese and yogurt*—cheese may be grated on soups or entrees. Use the reduced-fat varieties. (The fat-free cheeses often taste like rubber.) The best yogurt is fat free and organic without added fruit, but not frozen.

A **BIBLE CURE** *Health Fact*

God's Mediterranean Health Food: Olive Oil

Three basic types of olive oil work great for cooking and for pouring on salads or on pasta:

- *Extra-virgin olive oil:* I recommend using this kind of olive oil whenever possible. It's usually the purest and tastiest. Look at the color. The deeper the color, the more intense the olive flavor. Extra-virgin olive oil also has the most phytonutrients.
- *Pure or virgin olive oil:* It's paler than extra-virgin and is usually used for stir-frying in low heat.
- *Light olive oil:* This is often used for its healthy benefits, having the monounsaturated fats without the strong olive taste. "Light" refers to the oil's color and mildness of flavor, not its calorie count. It is more highly filtered to get this quality. It's also good for stir-frying at low temperatures.

Include the following foods in your Mediterranean diet a few times weekly:

- *Fish.* The healthiest fish are cold-water varieties such as cod, wild salmon, sardines, and tongol tuna. These are high in omega-3 fatty acids. One significant study in Europe found that lower cancer rates were associated with higher fish and fish oil consumption, whereas higher cancer rates came with increased animal fat consumption.[3]

- *Organic or free-range poultry.* Poultry should be eaten two to three times weekly. Eat white breast meat with the skin removed.

- *Organic or omega-3 eggs.* These should be eaten only in small amounts (two to three per week).

- *Organic or free-range lean red meat.* Red meat should be eaten only rarely, on an average of three times a month. (I suggest consuming less than 18 ounces of red meat a week.) Use only lean cuts with the fat trimmed. Use in small amounts as an additive to spice up soup or pasta. (Note: the severe restriction of red meat in the Mediterranean diet is a radical departure from the American diet, but it is a major contributor to the low rates of cancer and heart disease found in these countries.)

Why am I so particular about the types of meat I recommend? Cancer patients need adequate protein intake but not the toxic processed meats, such as bologna, bacon, sausage, or excessive amounts of red meat or pork. Instead, they need plant protein, such as beans, lentils, peas, legumes, nuts, seeds; healthy grains such as sprouted breads, wild or brown rice, millet, and others; organic eggs (two to three eggs with only one yolk), chicken, and turkey without the skin; wild salmon, sardines, and tongol tuna; and small amounts of organic, grass-feed beef. (Refer to my book *Eat This and Live!* for more information on healthy and unhealthy sources of protein.)

Why does protein matter so much? Cancer patients usually are in a negative nitrogen balance. When nitrogen intake equals nitrogen output, the person is in nitrogen balance, and this is the state of a healthy adult. Growing infants, children, and adolescents as well as pregnant women are in a positive nitrogen balance, which means more nitrogen is coming in than going out and the buildup of tissue is greater than the breakdown of tissue. A negative nitrogen balance occurs in cancer patients because their protein needs are increased.

Proteins are very important in forming the body's tissues, enzymes, hormones, antibodies, and other immune system components. Insufficient protein has a debilitating impact on the immune system. Cancer also interferes with the metabolism of protein by burning some of the body's protein for fuel, even if there is insufficient intake of protein and adequate intake of carbohydrates and fats to be used for energy. I encourage all of my cancer patients to take the amino acid supplement MAP and/or undenatured whey or plant protein supplements. (See Appendix A.)

Cooking methods are also very important to retain nutrient content in food and to minimize toxins. Stir-frying or steaming foods at lower temperatures rather than deep-frying or grilling—is being found to be healthier in study after study. When possible, choose organic foods grown as close as possible to where you live, which assures optimal nutritional value. Foods often lose their potency in the transit process, not to mention what they lose by having to be frozen or as they are bruised or buffeted from being bounced around in a freight train or in the back of a truck.

Whenever possible, meats should be cooked at lower temperatures (below 300 degrees and preferably around 250 degrees Fahrenheit). When meats are exposed to high temperatures, they produce chemicals not present in raw meats, and some of these are carcinogenic. Researchers have identified seventeen heterocyclic amines (HCAs), which appear as likely cancer encouragers, and these are not present in meats until they are cooked at higher temperatures. Studies have found that eating beef medium well to well done is linked to rates of stomach cancer three times higher than those who eat their beef rare or medium rare. While limiting meats will help with this, as will cooking at lower temperatures, grilling meats poses the largest concerns. So when you grill, use cancer-inhibiting spices such as turmeric or East Indian spice blends, and/or marinate your meats with red wine, berry juice, or cherry juice to counteract some of the HCA effects. Flipping your meats more often will also help lower the HCAs produced. Cooking thinner slices of meat at lower temperatures and marinating meats in red wine will reduce HCAs dramatically. Also be sure to cut off any char marks, which are toxic (and carcinogenic). Also, make sure you have lots of fresh fruits and veggies—and a good salad—to eat with your steaks or burgers!

Cold cuts and packaged meats like bologna, salami, hot dogs, bacon, sausage, and processed ham contain nitrites and nitrates, which may form cancer-causing chemicals called *nitrosamines* or *n-nitroso compounds*. These compounds are associated with cancer of the bladder, esophagus, stomach, brain, and oral cavity. If hot dogs are a favorite in your household, please switch to brands that say "nitrite-free" or "nitrate-free" on the label. Also, there are nitrite-free bacon, ham, sausage, and luncheon meats.

In addition, some extremely dangerous chemicals, such as DDT and PCBs, have been banned in the United States for decades, but since they remain in our water, land, and air, fish and animal products continue to be main sources of DDT and PCBs in our diets. The EPA lists DDT and PCBs as probable human carcinogens since both cause liver cancer in laboratory animals.[4]

These chemicals are stored in an animal's fat, so the best way to reduce your risk of ingesting DDT and PCBs is to choose lean cuts of organic meat and low-fat organic dairy products. Avoid predatory fish, which are often high in DDT and PCBs. Commercial fish that are high in PCBs include Atlantic and farmed salmon, bluefish, wild striped bass, white and Alantic croaker, blackback or winter flounder, summer flounder, and blue crab. Commercial fish that contain higher levels of pesticides, including DDT, are bluefish, wild striped bass, American eel, and Atlantic salmon.

Just as we benefit from following the Bible in moral conduct, we also benefit in following Bible directives on what we should eat. It is time for us to start letting the Bible change our minds about our diets as well as how we think and act.

> For the LORD your God is bringing you into a good land of flowing streams and pools of water, with fountains and springs that gush out in the valleys and hills. It is a land of wheat and barley; of grapevines, fig trees, pomegranates; of olive oil and honey.
> —DEUTERONOMY 8:7–8

This doesn't mean denying ourselves the things we love to eat so much as finding new things we like to replace old ones that, like sin, please us for a short time—only to try to kill us in the long run. It will take some counter-food-cultural living and changing the way we prepare meals; but, they are changes that could save your life down the road, so they are worth the self-control necessary to form new, healthier habits. Fruit and low-fat, low-sugar yogurts can replace ice cream and cake; fish and salad can replace beef and potatoes; and oranges, apples, berries, and pears or a handful of raw almonds, nuts, or seeds can fill in as snacks rather than candy bars or chips. Have Ezekiel 4:9 bread and almond butter rather than a peanut butter and jelly sandwich. You have to find what works for you and what you can stay with.

This is not a dietary change like cutting calories to lose weight, but it is something you need to start today and stick with for the rest of your life. So, think of it as a new adventure in following Jesus. Let it give a whole new meaning to the way you "break bread" with your friends and family!

A DEADLY BY-PRODUCT OF THE WESTERN DIET: INFLAMMATION

One of the biggest problems with our modern high-fat, highly processed, high-sugar, high-sodium diet is that it has thrown off the balance in our bodies between inflammatory and anti-inflammatory chemicals called *prostaglandins*. Normally, inflammation is a good thing that works to repair an injury or enables you to fight off infection in the body. It puts the immune system on high alert to attack invading bacteria or viruses to rid your body of these intruders. Or in the case of an injury, it rushes white blood cells to the cut, scrape, sprain, or broken bone to splint the injury and facilitate healing. This is the good side of inflammation and an extremely important function of the immune system's small agents. When our bodies are fighting an infection, there is a complicated process through which more pro-inflammatory prostaglandins are created than anti-inflammatory ones, and the immune system responds to the sounding of this alarm. When the crisis is over, the balance swings in the anti-inflammatory direction and eventually balances out again.

If you look at this process in a simplified sense, you will see that prostaglandins are produced from the foods we eat in an ongoing cycle, and each of the foods we eat has either a pro-inflammatory tendency or an anti-inflammatory one. Fatty acids are at the center of this. Omega-6 fatty acids are "friendly" to the creation of pro-inflammatory prostaglandins, and omega-3 fatty acids are "friendly" to the creation of anti-inflammatory prostaglandins. A more natural, Mediterranean-type diet will have a balance of pro- and anti-inflammatory-friendly foods; however, our modern high-fat, high-sodium, high-sugar, highly processed Western diet throws that balance off in favor of the production of pro-inflammatory prostaglandins.

Experts tell us that our typical U.S. diet has doubled the amount of omega-6 fatty acids we consume since 1940, as we have shifted more and more away from fruits and vegetables to grain-based foods and the oils produced from them. In fact, we eat about twenty times more omega 6s than we do the anti-inflammatory omega 3s. Humans today consume more cereal grains—and oils produced from them—than ever before in our history, and as a result we have more inflammatory diseases, including cancer, than ever before. Most of the animals we obtain food from today are also grain fed, so most of our meats, eggs, and dairy products are higher in omega-6 fats and more inflammatory than they were a century ago. Also, as most of the fish in our stores are now farm raised, they are growing up on cereal grains instead of the algae and smaller fish they would live on in the wild, so even our fish contain more omega-6 fats than they used to. Noting all of this, it is not hard to see why diseases caused by chronic systematic inflammation (including cancer) have grown to be such a problem in the Western world today.

Furthermore, omega-3 and omega-6 fats cannot be manufac-tured in the body and must be consumed either through diet or supplements. EFAs (essential fatty acids) help the body repair and create new cells. Thus omega-3 fat intake and the balance of different fats and oils are crucial for both preventing and limiting the spread of cancer. In addition to reducing inflamma-tion, omega-3 fatty acids can actually create special roadblocks in the body, making it harder for cancer cells to migrate from a primary tumor to start new colonies. Cancers that remain localized in one place are much easier to treat than those that metastasize (spread throughout the body).[5]

Patients with cancer are also more prone to have malabsorption and maldigestion, especially when undergoing chemotherapy. Malabsorption of fats is common in cancer patients, and fats and other important nutrients are not absorbed well. Maldigestion occurs when insufficient pancreatic enzymes and hydrochloric acid are produced. Both malabsorption and maldigestion usually cause weight loss and diarrhea, further weakening the immune system.

As we have seen, controlling inflammation is very important and is mainly done by balancing omega 6 fats and omega 3 fats. Research has shown that excessive dietary fat is associated with increased tumor growth. Also, when fat intake is decreased to 20 percent of calories from fat, natural killer cell activity is increased. All fats are not our enemy, but we need to learn to choose the good fats and avoid or limit the bad, inflammatory fats.

Cancer actually interferes with fat storage, as the body is less efficient in storing fat. This is one of the reasons most patients with advanced cancers look so thin and emaciated. Remember, fats help absorb the very important vitamin D3 and other fat-soluble vitamins, including vitamins A, E, and K. Adequate fat intake helps you maintain your protein so that your body doesn't burn protein as fuel. Fats are also the building blocks for cell membranes. Healthy fats include fatty fish, such as wild salmon; sardines; tongol tuna; anchovies; flax seeds; almonds; almond butter; macadamia nuts; avocados; guacamole; pecans; cashews; Brazil nuts; hazelnuts; olives; olive oil; avocado oil; macadamia nut oil, and flaxseed oil.

One may stir-fry at low heat with macadamia nut oil, olive

oil, or avocado oil; but, do not cook with flaxseed oil. Also, it's best to choose organic oils. These oils may also be added to smoothies to help you maintain your weight. One of my favorite smoothies for weight gain for cancer patients is to take 1 to 2 tablespoons of flaxseed oil with 1 to 2 tablespoons of olive oil and 1 scoop of undenatured whey or plant protein, 8 ounces of coconut kefir (or almond or skim milk), and ¼ cup of frozen berries. You may also add 1 to 2 tablespoons of ground-up flax-seeds or almond butter.

> O LORD, if you heal me, I will be truly healed; if you save me, I will be truly saved. My praises are for you alone!
>
> —JEREMIAH 17:14

Because of the high omega-6 content of our diets, our bodies produce more pro- rather than anti-inflammatory prostaglan-dins. Over time, the natural, ongoing creation of prostaglandins will tip the balance toward systematic inflammation as more pro-inflammatory prostaglandins are produced than anti-inflammatory ones. Despite the absence of an actual emergency, this imbalance still sets off alarms calling for inflammation, and the immune system will respond accordingly. However, with no actual threat present, the immune system may become confused and start attacking things it normally wouldn't. This immune hypersensitivity and chronic inflammation can lead to a glut of problems ranging from simple allergies and weight gain to cancer, Alzheimer's disease, cardiovascular disease, diabetes, arthritis, asthma, prostate problems, and autoimmune diseases.

Omega-3 fatty acids are clearly incredibly beneficial. Here are some omega-3 foods to include in your diet as a way to help prevent and battle cancer: flaxseeds and flaxseed oil, fish (wild salmon, tongal tuna, sardines, and anchovies), and pharmaceutical-grade fish oil. Obviously, it's important to know which fats to eat and which ones to avoid when it comes to preventing those harmful prostaglandins I mentioned above.

So, while using an understanding of the Mediterranean diet as a foundation, within that framework you should also look at how pro-inflammatory or anti-inflammatory the foods you eat are as well. Cancer is usually associated with chronic inflammation, and by eating more anti-inflammatory foods than pro-inflammatory ones, you can tip your balance back in the right direction.

One way to check your inflammation/anti-inflammation balance is by a blood test for C-reactive protein (CRP). C-reactive protein is simply a marker of inflammation, as well as a promoter of inflammation, and is one of the easiest indicators to test for. How high your CRP levels are will specify how significant your level of systematic inflammation is. Once you reach forty years of age, annual CRP testing is a great idea for checking the anti-inflammatory effectiveness of your diet.

A **BIBLE CURE** *Health Fact*

High CRP Levels Are *Not* Always a Danger Sign

Although elevated CRP levels are associated with an increased risk of cancer, remember that inflammation is a natural, healthy response to disease, and any infection or injury you suffer will temporarily raise your CRP levels to fight that crisis. Avoid having your CRP levels tested for at least two weeks after you have had an acute infection or suffered an injury to ensure your serum CRP level reflects your actual consistent level and hasn't been spiked due to some infection.

THE ANTI-INFLAMMATORY DIET: TAKING THE MEDITERRANEAN DIET TO THE NEXT LEVEL

So then, how do you escape this systemic inflammation that is causing cancer and so many health problems? First of all, you adopt the Mediterranean diet as the foundation for your day-in, day-out meal planning.

Then, within that framework, balance your pro-inflammatory and anti-inflammatory-friendly foods, and your CRP level will usually decrease accordingly. This will, of course, initially probably mean adding more anti-inflammatory foods and limiting or avoiding more pro-inflammatory ones for a time. I highly recommend Monica Reinagel's *The Inflammation-Free Diet Plan,* where she presents her years of research to ascribe an inflammation-free (IF) rating to the foods we eat. This rating system takes into account more than twenty different factors that contribute to a food's relationship to inflammation. Positive ratings are anti-inflammatory, and foods with negative ratings promote inflammation. Up to one hundred on each scale is considered mildly one way or the other, over one hundred is moderate, and over five hundred is severe.

Looking at her research and adding some of my own, I have organized the following two lists of foods for you to consider adding or subtracting from your diet as your level of systemic inflammation demands.

Top Anti-inflammatory Foods (Always Choose Organic When Possible and Do Not Deep-Fry)	
Fruit	Raspberries, acerola (West Indian) cherries, guava, strawberries, cantaloupe, lemons/limes, rhubarb, kumquat, pink grapefruit, mulberries
Vegetables	Chili peppers, onions (including scallions and leeks); spinach (greens, including kale, collards, turnip, and mustard greens); sweet potatoes; carrots; garlic
Legumes	Lentils, green beans
Egg Products	Liquid eggs, egg whites
Dairy	Cottage cheese (low fat and nonfat), nonfat cream cheese, plain yogurt (low fat and unsweetened), 1 ounce feta or part-skim mozzarella cheese, skim milk
Fish	Herring, mackerel (not king), wild salmon (not farmed; Alaskan preferred), rainbow trout, sardines, anchovies

Poultry (Remove Skin)	Goose, duck, free-range organic chicken and turkey (white meat)
Lean Meat (limit to 18 ounces or less per week)	Pot roast, beef shank, eye of round (beef), flank steak, sirloin tip, prime rib, skirt steak, pork rib chops*, pork tenderloin*, filet mignon, shellfish (including crab, lobster, and shrimp)*
Cereal	All-Bran, Total, bran flakes
Breads/ Pasta	Ezekiel 4:9 bread, sprouted breads, whole-wheat spaghetti (thick noodles), brown rice pasta, couscous, buckwheat groats, barley
Fats/Oils	Safflower oil (high oleic), hazelnut oil, olive oil, avocado oil, almond oil, apricot kernel oil, cod liver oil, macadamia nut oil, flaxseed oil (do not cook with this)
Nuts/Seeds	Brazil nuts, macadamia nuts, hazelnuts, pecans, almonds, hickory nuts, cashews, flaxseeds
Herbs/ Spices	Garlic, onion, cayenne, ginger, turmeric, chili peppers, chili powder, curry powder
Sweeteners	Stevia
Beverages	Carrot juice, tomato juice, black or green tea, club soda/seltzer, herbal tea, spring water

* The Bible states that this food was not intended to be eaten by men. If eating pork or shellfish concerns you for religious reasons, I recommend you avoid it. However, there is no scientific research to prove these foods are harmful if organic, free-range, lean selections are eaten in moderation.

Inflammatory Foods to Limit or Avoid	
Fruit	Mango, banana, dried apricots, dried apples, dried dates, canned fruits, raisins
Vegetables	Corn, white potatoes, french fries
Legumes	Baked beans, fava beans (boiled), canned beans
Egg Products	Duck eggs, goose eggs, hard-boiled eggs, egg yolks
Cheeses	Most all high-fat cheeses, including brick cheese, cheddar cheese, Colby cheese, cream cheese (normal and reduced fat)
Dairy	Flavored or fruit-on-the-bottom yogurt, ice cream, butter, whole milk, 2 percent milk, heavy whipping cream
Fish	Farmed salmon and other farm-raised fish, swordfish, tilefish, tuna, halibut, sea bass, bluefish, king mackerel
Poultry	Turkey (dark meat), Cornish game hen, chicken giblets, chicken liver, chicken (dark meat)
Meat	All processed meats and organ meats, bacon, all veal (loin and shank), pork chitterlings, all lamb (rib, chops, shanks, loin), pork ribs and shoulder roast
Breads	Hot dog/hamburger buns, English muffins, kaiser rolls, bagels, french bread, Vienna bread, blueberry muffins, oat bran muffins
Cereal	Grape-Nuts, Crispix, Corn Chex, Just Right, Rice Chex, corn flakes, Rice Krispies, Raisin Bran, shredded wheat

Pasta/Grain	White rice, millet, corn pasta, cornmeal, lasagna noodles, macaroni elbows, angel hair and regular spaghetti pasta
Fats/Oils	Margarine, wheat germ oil, sunflower oil, poppy seed oil, grape seed oil, safflower oil, cottonseed oil, palm kernel oil, coconut oil, corn oil
Nuts/Seeds	Poppy seeds, walnuts, pine nuts, sunflower seeds
Sweeteners	Honey, brown sugar, white sugar, corn syrup, powdered sugar, agave nectar
Crackers/ Chips/ Cookies	All cookies, chips, and crackers, including corn chips, pretzels, graham crackers, saltines, vanilla wafers, potato chips
Desserts	Sweetened-condensed milk, angel food cake, chocolate and vanilla cake with frosting, chocolate chips, whipped cream, ice cream, fruit leather snacks
Candy	All candy, including chocolate Kisses, jelly beans, Twix, Almond Joy, milk chocolate bars, Snickers
Beverages	All fruit juices and sodas, Gatorade, lemonade, sugar-laden soft drinks, commercial smoothies and coffees

These are not complete lists by any means—just some of the more likely "suspects" to watch out for or some of the more helpful foods to work into your diet. As you read these now, some of these will jump out at you as things you like and need, but you don't consume as much of them in your diet as you probably should. It is time to change your habits about certain foods and "lay them on the altar." The thing to remember is that you have a choice about what you put in your mouth, and now that you have a little more knowledge about these foods, you can begin making healthier diet choices concerning them.

CANCER IS LOSING THE BATTLE

Remember that something is constantly being done about the attacks on your healthy cells. Every minute of every day it's happening. While you are working, walking, eating, and relaxing, your body is already winning a silent war that is raging around and within you. It's because of your amazing immune system. This system, along with your white blood cells and vital organs, was wonderfully designed by God to overcome even the most powerful attacks by cancer-causing agents in foods and the environment. Be thankful that this incredible system is always at work to protect you.

Add to that the fact that you now also know something about how you can strengthen that immune system and keep it functioning at its peak efficiency. Diet directly impacts the immune system, either positively or negatively. Since your immune system is your body's first and strongest line of defense against cancer, you must be diligent to care for it and strengthen it by eating the right foods and avoiding harmful foods. What you eat makes all the difference!

> But he was pierced for our rebellion, crushed for our sins. He was beaten so we could be whole. He was whipped so we could be healed.
> —ISAIAH 53:5

A **BIBLE CURE** *Prayer for You*

*Lord, keep me mindful of the good things You have given
to us as food on this earth, and guide me and give me self-
discipline as I seek to transform my dietary habits. Give me
the willpower to overcome wrong cravings and the wisdom
to keep the wrong foods out of my house for the sake of my
family and our health. Link me with like-minded brothers
and sisters in my church family to help us stand together
to live healthy lives of blessing and giving to others.*

*Be close to me as I walk or exercise so that such times
can become times of fellowship with You. Remind me
constantly of what Your Word says about healing and
the plans You have for me to have a full and abundant life, one filled with health and a joyful heart.*

I pray this in the name of Jesus. Amen.

A **BIBLE CURE** *Prescription*

Healthy First Steps

You can begin to find hope for a better cancer-fighting immune system by taking these simple first steps today. Check off the ones you are now taking, and underline the ones you need to start immediately.

- ❏ Limit bad fats.
- ❏ Follow the Mediterranean diet.
- ❏ Avoid processed meats containing nitrites and nitrates.
- ❏ Eat more anti-inflammatory foods.
- ❏ Address your stress.
- ❏ Stop smoking.
- ❏ Stop worrying so much.
- ❏ Exercise regularly.
- ❏ Get eight hours of sleep per night.
- ❏ Consult your physician or a nutritional doctor.
- ❏ Pray for God's guidance and healing.

For more information on these topics, please read my book *The Seven Pillars of Health*.

Chapter 3

DR. COLBERT'S TOP SIXTEEN CANCER-FIGHTING AND -PREVENTING FOODS

I F YOU WANT to win the war against cancer, you'll need to eat the things that battle it. In the last chapter we looked at these more generally; now I'm going to fill this chapter with a description of your most powerful anticancer food allies so you can have no doubt about what to do. As you consider each one, please don't become overwhelmed, but begin to eat these foods a few days a week. Take one step at a time. Add the good things you are missing, and let go of the ones that have become harmfully habitual. Soon you'll realize that as your eating habits have been transformed, your body will follow.

> Have compassion on me, LORD, for I am weak. Heal me, LORD, for my bones are in agony.
>
> —PSALM 6:2

If this is your plea also, remember that God hears and answers. He also invites you to change for the better with His help, and He is clearly on your side.

There are numerous foods God has provided that go a long way in helping to prevent cancer, so I want to look at my top sixteen cancer-fighting and -preventing foods. Also, please note that cancers in different parts of the body often have very distinctly different natures, so foods that prevent one type of cancer do not necessarily have the same effects on others. For this reason I recommend consuming a variety of these powerful cancer-fighting foods a few times a week or on a daily basis. If you are looking for general cancer prevention, these foods are a great place to start.

1. BERRIES

Blueberries, strawberries, raspberries, black raspberries, cranberries, blackberries, and other berries have some of the highest antioxidant levels of any of the fruits. They are also excellent sources of several phytochemicals, which appear to inhibit cancer development. Ellagic acid is a powerful polypherol found especially in strawberries and raspberries. Anthocyanidins are a type of polypherol that is associated with the rich color pigments in berries, particularly blueberries and raspberries. The anthocyanidins and proanthocyanidins are key to the high antioxidant content of berries. While berries are typically only available during certain seasons, the most potent form of berries is freeze-dried, which should be available all year round and is great to sprinkle on salads, cereal, or in yogurt. Frozen berries are also a good alternative in smoothies or mixed with fresh yogurt as a cold dessert to replace ice cream. It's best to choose organic berries since berries are prone to contain pesticide residues.

Researchers at Ohio State University did a series of experiments to test the anticarcinogenic effects of black raspberries on cancer in rats. The experiments were done by feeding rats a carcinogen, and then the experimental groups were fed a diet of 5 and 10 percent powdered black raspberries. These amounts reduced the number of esophageal cancer tumors that developed at fifteen weeks by 39 and 49 percent respectively. After twenty-five weeks, however, the average results for the respective groups were a 62 and 43 percent reduction, suggesting that you can overdo it. According to researcher Gary D. Stoner, PhD, "The National Cancer Institute recommends that every American eat at least four to six helpings of fruit and vegetables each day. We suggest that one of these helpings be berries of some sort."[1] Include different types of berries, including strawberries, blueberries, raspberries, blackberries, and cranberries, etc., instead of the juice.

2. CRUCIFEROUS VEGETABLES

Cruciferous vegetables contain a host of cancer-preventive agents (also called *chemopreventive agents*) that act in various ways to block cancer development at its most critical stages. There is a good deal of evidence now that higher consumption of cruciferous vegetables is directly associated with lower rates of different cancers, especially in the colon, prostate, lungs, or breasts.

Cruciferous vegetables also contain *benzyl isothiocyanate* (BITC, read "bit-c"). BITC encourages apoptosis (programmed cell death) in breast cancer cells by interfering with their ability to use energy. In ovarian cancer cells, BITC stimulates the cellular signals that inform the cancer that it is time to shut down and die. Either of these "arrests" in the cell cycle of cancer will prevent or shrink tumors. Many drugs used in chemotherapy have basically this same aim, but they will interrupt the function of normal cells as well as cancer cells. Since breast cancer cells are more susceptible to this arrest, BITC will usually trigger the apoptosis of these cells without affecting healthy cells, something chemotherapy cannot do.

Furthermore, BITC inhibits cancer promotion by hindering cytochrome enzymes from acting on initiated cells, and thus is a great cancer preventative.[2] This compound also inhibits cancer-promoting estrogen receptors in breast cancer. BITC sensitizes pancreatic cells to radiation therapy, potentially increasing its effectiveness and reducing the dosages of radiation needed for treatment. It also increases the production of reactive oxygen species in pancreatic cancer, contributing to their destruction. (Cancers do not do well in oxygen-rich tissues.) This is ground-breaking news, as pancreatic cancer is particularly treatment resistant and deadly.

The *indole-3-carbinol* (I3C) also found in cruciferous vegetables helps promote detoxification as well as blocks the activation of carcinogens. I3C converts into *diindolylmethane* (DIM) in the GI tract, a compound that contributes to immune system function, discourages angiogenesis (the formation of new blood vessels cancer will use to siphon nutrients from the blood), and promotes apoptosis in prostate and breast cancer cells. DIM also seems to complement the effects of standard chemotherapy agents even in strains of cancer that have historically been treatment resistant.

Because of the power of these different compounds and others found in broccoli, cauliflower, watercress, cabbage, kale, brussels sprouts, and the like, they have long been at the top of the list of cancer-fighting foods. Extracts from these are also readily available today, though your mother's advice is still solid: "Honey, eat your broccoli—it's good for you!" Consider taking

OncoPLEX, which is a capsule containing broccoli sprouts. (See Appendix A.)

3. GREEN TEA

Laboratory research has shown time and again that green tea catechins, including *epigallocatechin-3 gallate* (EGCG), reduce the growth of various kinds of cancer cells. A landmark study presented in 2005 by researchers from two Italian universities recently demonstrated that green tea catechins were 90 percent effective in keeping men with premalignant lesions in the prostate from developing prostate cancer.[3] In fact, more than 135 different studies have supported the claim that ingesting certain levels of green tea helps to fight cancer.

EGCG is readily absorbed into the body and has been shown to promote cancer cell apoptosis and prevent angiogenesis, and it has important antioxidant properties. It has also been shown with *epicatechin-3 gallate* (ECG)—another component of green tea—to indirectly lower the synthesis of dihydrotestosterone (DHT), which has been identified as an accomplice in contributing to prostate cancer and enlargement. Researchers at the University of Rochester in New York also recently announced that EGCG targets heat shock protein 90, a protein present in cancer cells more than normal cells.[4] This protein makes the cells resistant to chemotherapy and radiation therapy, so EGCG shows promise in thwarting the growth and survival of cancer cells already under treatment.

> My child, pay attention to what I say. Listen carefully to my words. Don't lose sight of them. Let them penetrate deep into your heart, for they bring life to those who find them, and healing to their whole body.
>
> —PROVERBS 4:20–22

Green tea catechins also appear to have chemopreventive effects on colon, rectal, lung, stomach, and kidney cancers as well as prostate cancer. Research has long shown that cultures that drink a good deal of green tea, such as several in Asia, have lower incidences of various kinds of cancer. In fact, despite Japan's high smoking rate, its rates of lung cancer remain consistently lower than Western countries.[5] Japanese green tea contains significantly more EGCG than Chinese green tea. Green tea's benefits also include fighting cardiovascular disease, obesity, and osteoporosis. Green tea is a great substitute for coffee; you can also add green tea extract to your daily supplement routine.

4. FISH OIL

As we discussed in the last chapter, the omega-3 fatty acids found in fish oil are both lacking in the typical Western diet, and getting them through eating a large amount of cold-water fish can be potentially dangerous because of the increased levels of mercury commonly found in fish today. Because of this, pharmaceutical-grade fish oil capsules are almost universally recommended as a supplement every westerner should have in their daily regimen.

Various studies have tied the high consumption of fish in

areas like Sweden and Japan to lower rates of prostate and breast cancers in those areas.[6] It has also been linked to preventing colon cancer.[7] It is believed that omega 3s do this by decreasing inflammation and the DNA damage that can inspire mutations, enhancing DNA repair, and encouraging cancer cell apoptosis.

One word of caution, however: not all nutritional supplements are created equal. In the same way that people will strip-mine the countryside for a metal or cut corners manufacturing a product, producers have looked for so many ways to cut the costs on these supplements that few are of high enough quality to give you the proper benefits. Fish oil capsules are among the worst violators of quality control. Pharmaceutical-grade products have been tested for heavy metals and other toxins. However, some still contain rancid fish oils. For this reason I ask patients to bring in their fish oil capsules so that I can examine them. I usually will stick a hypodermic needle in them, draw out some of the oil, put a drop on their finger, and have them taste it. Typically they will grimace and say, "Why did you make me do that? That stuff's awful!"

The reason is that the fish oils in their supplement are usually rancid. This happens far too often. Taste yours for yourself to see. If these oils are rancid, they can be worse than taking no omega-3 oils at all, because the rancid oils will produce free radicals, among which is the particularly dangerous lipid free radical hydroperoxide, which is linked to very serious diseases, including cancer. Do your research on whatever you are taking as supplements, and make sure you are getting what you need in what you are paying for. (See Appendix A.)

5. PARSLEY, CELERY, AND ARTICHOKES

Parsley, celery, and artichokes contain low concentrations of a phytochemical called *apigenin*. Apigenin inhibits angiogenesis in ovarian cancer cells, which, as you will likely remember, is the process by which tumors instruct the body to build new blood vessels to reach to wherever they happen to have latched on to an organ so that they can feed themselves. Preventing angiogenesis keeps the cancer cells from hijacking the body's food supply for itself and stymies its growth and ability to spread. Apigenin interferes with cancer cells' ability to burn glucose in the pancreas, another important function that starves cancers. Apigenin is also an anti-inflammatory agent, and, as if that weren't enough, it also promotes apoptosis *within* tumors, shrinking them and heading others off before they even have a chance to form. A 2009 study from Harvard's Channing Laboratory found that of five different flavonoids, only apigenin was associated with a significant reduction in cancer risk.[8] Thus adding these vegetables to your diet is another way to get God's natural healers hidden in our foods.

6. SPROUTS—BROCCOLI, WHEAT, ETC.

Broccoli sprouts are high in *sulforaphane*, which contributes to the detoxification of carcinogens, promotes apoptosis, interrupts cancer cell replication, makes healthy tissue more tumor resistant, fights metastasis, and blocks the cancer-producing effects of exposure to ultraviolet radiation. According to Johns Hopkins University's Paul Talalay, "Three-day-old broccoli sprouts consistently contain 20 to 50 times the amount of chemoprotective compounds found in mature broccoli heads, and may offer a simple, dietary means of chemically reducing cancer risk."[9] Broccoli sprouts (or teas made from them) appear to be especially high in these cancer-defeating compounds.

While broccoli sprouts have gotten most of the press because of the studies done on them, clover and alfalfa sprouts are high in phytoestrogens, which, as we have already seen, are important in preventing breast and prostate cancers. Alfalfa sprouts and wheat sprouts are also high in antioxidants and phytonutrients. It appears that "sprouting" these vegetables gives them increased benefits because many of their phytonutrients are very potent in the seeds that are only a few days old. Wheat sprouts are high in chlorophyll and also contain chlorophyllin, a powerful phytonutrient that blocks aflatoxin, a carcinogenic fungus that grows on grains such as corn and rice. It also blocks heterocyclic amines, which are carcinogenic. As one expert in the field, Gabriel Cousens, put it, "Sprouts contain a rainforest of undiscovered and known good health characteristics such as antioxidants, anti-carcinogens, live enzymes, high levels of vitamins, nucleic acids, paciferans (plant antibiotics), auxones (beneficial plant hormones), and other factors."[10] If you are not into sprouting, consider taking OncoPLEX, which is a capsule containing broccoli sprouts. (See Appendix A.)

7. TURMERIC

Turmeric is a yellow-brown spice obtained from powdering the dried stalk of a plant in the ginger family found primarily in India and Indonesia. Since turmeric is highly present in the diets of these countries and they have a significantly lower incidence of cancer (which is roughly a third of the incidence in the United States),[11] many are pointing to it as a potentially wonderful preventative for various types of cancer. Though more study is needed on turmeric itself to determine all of its anticarcinogenic properties, it is a highly anti-inflammatory food (and inflammation is at the root of many cancers). Aside from that, however, turmeric's primary active ingredient is curcumin, which is what gives turmeric its brilliant yellow color. It also appears that curcumin has powerful therapeutic properties on its own.

Curcumin is an antioxidant several times more powerful than vitamin E and works to inhibit the formation of blood clots, and naturally lowers cholesterol. It appears to be a very promising agent for preventing skin cancer, as well as an inhibitor of nuclear factor-kappa beta (NFkB), a protein complex that seems to play an important role in the life cycle of cancer cell development. By interfering with the function of NFkB, curcumin promotes apoptosis in the cancer cells that form in the skin, prostate, breasts, cervix, colon, and lungs, as well as in leukemia and multiple myeloma.

One hurdle for curcumin consumption is that it is hard for our digestive tract to absorb it into the bloodstream. To the rescue for this is piperine, a molecule found in pepper that increases the absorption of curcumin by about one thousand times. Perhaps the reason curcumin has been so beneficial in India and Indonesia is that pepper and turmeric are normally combined together in most curry powders and sauces. Thus, adding a teaspoon of turmeric to soups, salad dressings, and pasta dishes that also contain pepper is a great way to get incredible anticarcinogenic power in a small, tasty package.

8. GARLIC AND ONIONS

Garlic and onions contain phytochemical compounds that appear particularly good at keeping the nitrates and nitrites in our foods from converting into nitrosamines, a class of compounds with numerous cancer-causing characteristics. Because of this, these seem particularly effective in preventing esophageal, stomach, and colon cancers. Nitrates are particularly high in pickled foods and processed or cured meats such as sausage, bacon, and ham. While vegetables also contain some nitrates, these seem to be counteracted by the vitamin C they also contain; thus these plant nitrates do not turn into toxic compounds. Garlic appears to have a greater protective power than onions, but onions are far more prevalent in most Western diets. Crushed fresh garlic seems to have the highest amount of cancer-fighting compounds.

Besides these preventative qualities, molecules found in these vegetables also appear to slow the spread of tumors and encourage apoptosis through interfering with the growth process of cancer cells. While more study is needed to determine how exactly compounds in garlic and onions have these effects, there is enough evidence now available to suggest that adding these *allium* family vegetables to spice up our foods is a wise step toward an anticancer diet plan.

9. POMEGRANATE

Studies continue to reinforce that pomegranate—eaten, drank as a juice, or taken in extract form—has incredible anti-inflammatory properties, increases antioxidants in the blood, and inhibits hormone-driven cancers. Pomegranate is chocked full of *ellagitannins*, which appear to interfere with the hormonal cycles that promote breast and prostate cancers. As it is digested, pomegranate also releases ellagic acid, a compound we have already discussed in the cancer-fighting attributes of berries. Research is still being done on this wonder fruit, but with pomegranates' ability to fight other illnesses as well, such as arthritis and heart disease, it is worth considering adding a daily glass (2 to 4 ounces) of pomegranate juice to your normal breakfast routine. A study conducted by UCLA researchers found that drinking 8 ounces of pomegranate juice a day decreased prostate cancer, doubling time from fifteen months to fifty-four months.

10. TOMATOES

Tomatoes are the best dietary source of the carotenoid lycopene, which is the substance that gives tomatoes their bright red color. However, unlike many other vegetables (or fruits, if you want to be absolutely correct about it), tomatoes are not best eaten in their raw form. Tomato paste is richest in lycopene, while spaghetti sauces, ketchup, and tomato sauce have roughly half as much as the paste they are made from. From there, tomato soup, canned tomatoes, and tomato juice all have about a third the lycopene that tomato paste has. Raw tomatoes have a little over 10 percent the lycopene of tomato paste.

There are a number of studies that have tied lycopene with a reduced risk of prostate cancer, though these results have not been universally proven in all the research done on the relationship. The benefits of lycopene-rich diets, however, seem most beneficial in the men most at risk for prostate cancer, those age sixty-five and above. It seems lycopene corrects something the aging process weakens. However, tomatoes are also an excellent source of antioxidants, so they further counteract the effects of systematic inflammation. Research continues on the exact reasons that tomatoes aid in the fight against prostate cancer, but the correlation is strong enough and there are enough other health benefits from sauces made from tomatoes that adding tomato products to your diet is a smart move. Eating something with tomato sauce in it as little as twice a week is thought to lower the risk of prostate cancer by around 25 percent.[12]

11. FLAXSEED AND LIGNANS

Flaxseed is one of the richest sources of plant lignans that act as plant hormones and inhibit the effects of testosterone and estrogen on hormone-sensitive cancers like those in the prostate and breasts. These lignans work to alter estrogen metabolism, block angiogenesis, and encourage apoptosis in these cancers. In a recent study of three thousand women, eleven hundred of whom had confirmed cases of breast cancer, researchers deduced that premenopausal women with a high lignan intake reduced their risk of cancer by about 44 percent.[13] One of these flaxseed lignans, *enterolactone*, was found in another study to have "a strong protective effect on breast cancer risk."[14] Another study found that men with the highest levels of enterolactone were 82 percent less likely to have prostate cancer.[15]

Flaxseed can be added to your diet either whole or ground up and put into soups, onto salads, into smoothies, or by any of a number of similar ways. Flaxseed oil does not have the high lignan content that flaxseeds do.

12. CITRUS AND QUERCETIN

While citrus fruits are famous for their vitamin C, a valuable antioxidant linked to all kinds of wonderful benefits, these fruits are also among the best sources available of flavones, as well as fiber, folic acid, and potassium. These fruits also contain limonoids, which have been shown to have powerful anticancer characteristics. Since these are not found in any other fruit except citrus, this makes their cancer-fighting potential unique.

Most think primarily of oranges, lemons/limes, and grapefruit when you mention citrus fruits. However, you should also consider adding foods high in vitamin C, such as pineapples, tomatoes, kumquats, mandarin oranges, and tangerines to your diet for variety. Studies from around the world have time and again linked the consumption of citrus fruits (not juices) with a decreased risk of developing different cancers, especially those of the digestive tract: esophageal, mouth, larynx, pharynx, and stomach. Results varied, but most showed a decrease of 40 to 50 percent.[16]

One of the most powerful flavonoids found in citrus fruit is *quercetin*. Research over the years has shown quercetin to stimulate the immune system's ability to tear apart tumors, salvage free radicals, inhibit the division of cancer cells, prohibit cell mutation, lessen angiogenesis, and encourage apoptosis. *Citrus pectin* (a polysaccharide found in the cell wall of citrus fruit) has been shown to decrease metastases in animal studies of prostate cancer and melanoma.[17]

Again, while further study is needed to fathom the full depth of anticancer potency in these fruits, there is certainly enough evidence that citrus should be an important component of the fruits and vegetables that you eat on a daily basis for all of their health benefits. I prefer that my patients consume lemons and limes squeezed in a glass of water and drink it throughout the day. These citrus fruits are low glycemic and also very alkanizing to the tissues. I will be talking about the importance of alkanizing the tissues later in this book.

13. RED GRAPES, RED WINE, AND RESVERATROL

Resveratrol, a polyphenol found in red grapes and red wines, is a natural protective agent that makes grapes resilient to attacks by microorganisms. As a rule, resveratrol is in the skins and seeds of the grapes, which are left in much longer during the fermentation process for red wines than for white; therefore red wines have higher levels of this valuable compound. Grapes that are grown in harsher climates also seem to have higher levels of resveratrol than those grown in more temperate areas. It seems the more the grapes suffer, the better they are for us.

Since the resveratrol resides in the skins and seeds, it is not as easily absorbed into our bodies in the raw form as it is when the grapes are crushed and fermented whole into red wine. In fact, the fermentation process for red wine also makes it rich in polyphenols. Red wines are probably the most complex beverages in the human diet because of all the different molecules in them. The bottling process for wines help preserve the resveratrol, while other things that come from grapes, like raisins, have had almost all of the resveratrol leeched out of them.

For those who don't want the alcohol also present in red wines, there are nonalcoholic alternatives you can find in most health food stores and resveratrol capsules. (See Appendix A.) Grape and cranberry juices also have resveratrol in them, but at about a tenth the level of red wines and contain too much sugar. Resveratrol supplements such as Living Resveratrol will give you the resveratrol of six hundred glasses of red wine without having to drink any. Such supplements are often extracted from ground-up Japanese knotweed, which is remarkably high in resveratrol as well. If choosing grapes or red wine, it's best to choose organic.

> Don't worry about anything; instead, pray about everything. Tell God what you need, and thank him for all he has done.
>
> —PHILIPPIANS 4:6

Resveratrol was the first natural nutrient to have significant evidence behind it as a cancer preventative and one that will arrest cancer right in its footsteps. Resveratrol has been proven effective in reducing the risk and/or growth of breast, prostate, colon, skin, pancreatic, ovarian, liver, lung, stomach, oral, cervical, lymphatic, thyroid, and esophageal cancers, as well as melanoma, leukemia, metastasis to bones, and neuroblastoma.[18] Research is also being done on its ability to boost the effects of chemotherapy and to do its work without harming normal, noncancerous cells.

14. SOY

Hormone-driven cancers such as breast and prostate cancers seem to be encouraged by excess estrogen or testosterone in our bodies, but they appear to be inhibited by the presence of *phytoestrogens* such as those found in many products that are made from soybeans. Phytoestrogens (*phyto-* is a Greek root word meaning "plant") are only about one one-thousandth as strong as normal estrogen and will "lock into the place" of estrogen on certain cancer-promoting molecules, thus decreasing the tumor-promoting effects of those agents. So, soy's phytoestrogens actually inhibit the ability of cancer cells to reproduce themselves and grow into tumors.

Soy also contains anticarcinogenic *isoflavones*. In a study of men from Japan, China, and the United States, it was demonstrated that legumes like soy reduced the incidence of prostate cancer by 38 percent, that eating yellow-orange vegetables reduced it by 33 percent, and that eating cruciferous vegetables reduced it by 39 percent, even across the various ethnicities.[19] Another study linked the eating of tofu once a week with a 15 percent decrease in the risk of breast cancer in women.[20]

As a rule, Asian women who eat soy most of their lives get several benefits that reduce their breast cancer risk. *Genistein*, an isoflavone found in soybeans, promotes the formation of differentiated tissue in the breasts, making it harder for any one kind of cancer to get a firm foothold. It also increases the density of breast cells, making early detection of a potential tumor much easier. Genistein also protects against the metastasis of prostate cancer cells and helps prevent angiogenesis, as well as protecting an anticancer vitamin D metabolite.

In a study using mice, subjects were fed three different soy products: soy protein without isoflavones, a soy-phytochemical concentrate including a number of compounds (one of which was genistein), and genistein alone. The genistein-only group had a 57 percent reduction in tumor growth, and the phytochemical concentrate groups saw a 70 percent reduction. The soy-phytochemical group also saw a halt in metastasis in the lymph nodes and lungs, as well as increased apoptosis and inhibited angiogenesis.[21] Soy isoflavones also appear to block the spreading of prostate cancer, modulate hormone promotion of the disease, interrupt the signals of the cancer cells' development cycle, encourage their apoptosis, and may even activate and deactivate cancer-related genes. Genistein also appears to affect non-hormone-driven cancers by inhibiting tyrosine kinase (TK), which promotes the formation and spread of new cancer cells.

> Then if my people who are called by my name will humble themselves and pray and seek my face and turn from their wicked ways, I will hear from heaven and will forgive their sins and restore their land.
> —2 CHRONICLES 7:14

However, a person doesn't have to search too widely on the Internet today to find that soy is coming under attack and that it may not be the cure-all some have tried to make it. One of the main issues is that most soy products are made from soybeans that have been genetically modified, and a growing field of research pointing to the potential dangers of genetically modified (GMO) foods. In a recent study, hamsters fed on genetically modified soy lost the ability to reproduce and experienced higher levels of infant mortality.[22]

As with any product that comes into wider demand, the industry response is to provide it in larger quantities and different forms. However, this raises some concerns. For instance, using soy-based baby formulas promotes very high phytoestrogen levels in infants for no scientifically valid reasons, and many are now beginning to feel this may be harmful. One certain strand of breast cancer, MCF-7, appears to actually be promoted by genistein rather than inhibited by it, so further questions have arisen about the benefits of soy. (Note that studies on this are in their infancy and that it has been shown that MCF-7 breast cancer cells already have to be present for genistein to promote them; it will not encourage their initial development.) Certainly this makes adding soy to your diet worth discussing with your personal physician, but soy still seems to be very beneficial for men with prostate cancer, especially if you can find it in a form that has not been genetically modified. Edamame (soybeans), miso, dry roasted soybeans, tofu, and soy flour are good sources of soy isoflavones. Soy milk, soy sauce, and soy oil are very low in isoflavones.

15. CILANTRO

Coriander is a European herb in the parsley family. Its leaves are known as cilantro (or Chinese parsley). Cilantro leaves help flush out heavy metals by accelerating the excretion of lead, cadmium, asbestos, mercury, and aluminum through the urine, making it an inexpensive way to chelate toxic metals from the body. Dr. Yoshiaki Omura, an oncologist, has been treating patients with breast cancer, lung cancer, colon cancer, and prostate cancer with a method in which he combines the use of cilantro with one of many drug-uptake enhancement methods by pressing firmly on acupuncture points.

According to Dr. Omura, drug uptake can be inhibited by synthetic clothing, bras, necklaces, earrings, watches whose batteries are oriented with the positive side facing the body, and metal bands or bracelets. Dr. Omura also examines patients' bedrooms for the possibility of invisible but harmful electromagnetic fields, which he believes can contribute to cancer as well.

I recommend that you order cilantro tablets from Dr. Omura (see Appendix A), especially if you cannot tolerate the taste of cilantro. For those who enjoy the taste, I also recommend using the fresh cilantro herb in salads, soups, salsas, tacos, or as a garnish with any dish.

16. CHOCOLATE

When it comes to chocolate, the darker the better, because the darker the chocolate, the higher the cacao concentration. Though cacao beans are roughly 50 to 57 percent fat, the good fats (oleic acid, a monounsaturated fat also found in olive oil) outweigh the bad in dark chocolate, so it is neutral in its effect on blood cholesterol. The same is not true of milk chocolate. Dark chocolate has a relatively low glycemic index, but it depends on its sugar content. Because of these attributes, if eaten in moderation, dark chocolate can be an enhancer of healthy desserts, such as berries, or part of a high-energy snack.

The reason dark chocolate could be worth its calories (other than just its taste) is that it is full of polyphenols. Fifty grams of dark chocolate has more polyphenols than a cup of green tea and about twice that of a glass of red wine. Chocolate also contains proanthocyanidins. Research has found that the proanthocyanidins can slow the progress of certain cancers (particularly lung cancer) and inhibit angiogenesis. Though more research is needed to confirm these findings, there is growing evidence that these proanthocyanidins interfere with several events in the formation and progression of cancers, thus tripping it up and slowing it down enough for a healthy immune system to deal with easily.

However, remember this is with moderation, as is true with red wine (best limited to one glass a day). An ounce and a half of dark chocolate a day should give you the maximum benefit from this "luxury food" without tipping the balance in the wrong direction because of its high sugar and fat contents. Do not choose milk chocolate but rather dark chocolate containing at least 70 percent cocoa mass (such as Dagoba chocolate), and make sure it is low in sugar.

DEFUSING THE RISK FACTORS

What a powerful person is our Lord Jesus Christ, and what a wonderful creation the Father has provided for us so full of wonderful things to eat that will also give us long and healthy lives! What great compassion God has used in exercising His power. Read through the Gospels, and you'll see Jesus going from place to place, constantly offering healing and forgiveness to all who approached Him. One of my favorite accounts is this story of healing from a truly dreaded disease:

> Large crowds followed Jesus as he came down the mountainside. Suddenly, a man with leprosy approached him and knelt before him. "Lord," the man said, "if you are willing, you can heal me and make me clean." Jesus reached out and touched him. "I am willing," he said. "Be healed!" And instantly the leprosy disappeared.
>
> —MATTHEW 8:1–3

Healing people is still God's desire today. Have you approached Him lately for His healing? For His compassion? For His power? He is ready to give you all these good things, through His supernatural power when needed, but more often through just His day-to-day wisdom for living lives reflecting His compassion to the world. If we are crippled by sickness or cancer—especially if it is because we have been negligent of the abundance of good things He has given us to eat to keep us strong and full of life—what kind of testimony are we to such a loving God? I want to assure you that the Lord has already with great compassion built into our foods a good amount of power too—healing and cancer-fighting power! It is up to us, however, to work them into our diets and have the self-control to stay away from the things that will harm us—and those we will discuss in the next chapter.

A **BIBLE** **CURE** *Prayer for You*

Father, I thank You so much for all of the wonderful things You have given us on this earth, especially the bountiful foods full of nutritional and healing power. Help me to crave these good foods just as I crave to please You in my daily walk and lifestyle upon the earth. Let me never take for granted the wonderful things You have given to us for our health and fullness of life.

I thank You in the name above every name,
Jesus Christ, the great Healer. Amen.

A BIBLE CURE *Prescription*

Choosing Your Power Foods

Are you eating your power foods? From the list below, check the ones you eat regularly, and circle those you need to start adding to your diet NOW!

❏ Artichoke
❏ Broccoli
❏ Broccoli sprouts
❏ Brussels sprouts
❏ Black currants
❏ Black raspberries
❏ Blueberries
❏ Cabbage
❏ Cauliflower
❏ Celery
❏ Cold-water fish
❏ Cranberries
❏ Dark chocolate (1½ ounces)
❏ Flaxseed
❏ Garlic
❏ Grapefruit
❏ Green tea
❏ Kale
❏ Kumquats
❏ Lemons/limes

❏ Mandarin oranges
❏ Mixed greens
❏ Onions
❏ Oranges
❏ Parsley
❏ Pineapple
❏ Pomegranate (or its juice)
❏ Raspberries
❏ Red grapes
❏ Red wine (or extract)
❏ Strawberries
❏ Tangerines
❏ Tofu
❏ Tomatoes
❏ Turmeric (curry powder)
❏ Watercress
❏ Wheat sprouts

Chapter 4

CANCER-FEEDING FOODS TO AVOID

WHEN KING DAVID experienced healing from the hand of God, he lifted his heart in praise, declaring, "O LORD my God, I cried out to you for help, and you restored my health" (Ps. 30:2). I hope that you too are lifting your heart daily to the Lord—yes, crying out to Him for help whenever you need it. You don't even have to use words, for as Victor Hugo once said, "Certain thoughts are prayers. There are moments when, whatever be the attitude of the body, the soul is on its knees."[1]

As you seek the Lord in your thoughts and prayers, remember that the restoration of health, from a medical point of view, usually involves some kind of detoxification of the body to make way for the restoration of healthy processes. There are just things we don't need in our systems, and a great place to start is by avoiding—or at least minimizing—the intake of foods that have been proven to be cancer encouraging rather than cancer defeating.

CANCER: THE JUNK-FOOD JUNKIE

As a whole, cancers are sugar feeders; they feed on sugars. When you choose to eat sugar, you are giving cancer its favorite food. Cancer cells have metabolisms as much as eight times higher than those of normal cells, so the quick burst of hyper-energy provided by high levels of glucose in your bloodstream create a very fertile environment for cancers to develop, grow, and spread. In fact, one of the early detection methods now being used to locate tumors is to inject the patient with radioactive glucose and then give them a positron emission tomography (PET) scan. Since a tumor will gobble up sugar in the blood, any tumors appear as bright, white splotches on the PET scan images. Individuals without tumors will have no such spots.

Add to that the fact that high sugar levels also impede immune system functions and fan the flames of inflammation, and suddenly sugar becomes a double ally of cancer. So, step one for any cancer diet is to reduce your sugar intake and to avoid or limit high-glycemic foods, both of which feed cancer.

The glycemic index (GI) gives an indication of the rate at which different carbs and foods break down to release sugar in the bloodstream. High-glycemic foods are foods that raise the blood sugar rapidly. The University of Sydney manages a Web site at www.glycemicindex.com that allows you to search foods and see their glycemic index rating. The faster a food is converted to sugar, the more rapidly the blood sugar rises and the higher the glycemic index. Processed foods and those high in refined carbohydrates usually have higher GIs. Foods that have a glycemic index of 55 or under are considered low glycemic. Non-starchy vegetables will typically have a GI rating hovering around 0 to 1. The glycemic index is only for carbohydrates and not for fats and proteins. Sugars and carbohydrates that are digested rapidly, such as white bread, white rice, and instant potatoes, raise the blood sugar rapidly and have a GI of 70 or higher. Foods such as beans, peas, lentils, sweet potatoes and other green veggies are digested slowly and release sugars gradually in the bloodstream.

They are considered low glycemic, with a GI of 55 or lower. For more information on the glycemic index, please see my book *Dr. Colbert's "I Can Do This" Diet*.

Ingesting soluble fiber before your meals or eating foods high in fiber will lower the glycemic index of the food, as will cooking with healthy oils such as olive oil, macadamia nut oil, and so forth.

Here's a rule of thumb for this if you don't have a way to search the Web for the actual glycemic index number: judge by color. White foods (white bread, white sugar, white rice, baked potatoes, white pastas, etc.) tend to be higher on the glycemic index scale than colorful fruits and vegetables—sweet potatoes, beans, peas, lentils, and Ezekiel 4:9 bread. In order not to feed cancer, it's best to avoid refined sugars, refined flours, and artificial sweeteners also (especially foods and beverages that contain aspartame, which has its own links to cancer). Darker chocolate is better than lighter chocolate. While this may not be universally true, it is at least something to keep in the back of your mind when you are out eating or traveling.

According to a recent study, there is evidence that cancer cells also need glutamine, an amino acid, to utilize glucose, and that in the absence of glutamine, glucose will go unused.[2] This research may lead to possibilities for new glutamine-blocking drugs for cancer treatment. However, normal and cancer cells both need glutamine and glucose to function, so as a normal dietary concern for someone without cancer, you are better off decreasing your sugar intake by avoiding high glycemic foods and sugar than you are worrying about your glutamine levels. Also, many cancer patients are in negative nitrogen balance or protein deficient, and limiting glutamine will encourage this.

One day while Jesus was teaching, some Pharisees
and teachers of religious law were sitting nearby.
(It seemed that these men showed up from every
village in all Galilee and Judea, as well as from
Jerusalem.) And the Lord's healing power was
strongly with Jesus.

—LUKE 5:17

In this category, sodas of all kinds are big violators, even if
they are not sweetened with high-fructose corn syrup. Artificial sweeteners appear to be just as bad as sugars, if not worse.
A recent study estimated that individuals who consume two or
more soft drinks a week have an 87 percent higher risk of pancreatic cancer than those who don't. Further research into this is
needed, however, as drinking soft drinks is somewhat difficult
to separate from other harmful elements such as smoking,
caloric intake, being overweight, and having type 2 diabetes,
since many who drink a lot of soft drinks also participate in one
or more of these activities as well.[3]

Unsweetened iced teas and soda or seltzer waters are good
replacements, and remember to add a squeeze of lemon or lime.
Natural vegetable juices—especially if you are making them at
home with your own juicer—are wonderful options, especially
since they have the added benefit of detoxifying the body, but
add 1 to 2 tablespoons of the pulp back to the juice. Probably the
best way to get the highest dose of carotenoids is to drink a half
to a full cup of fresh carrot juice. I usually do this a few days a
week in the midmorning. Processing carrots in a juicer makes a
perfect carrot cocktail. The juicer breaks apart the carrot's fibers,
releasing the beta-carotene. (Again, just remember to add 1 to

2 tablespoons of pulp back to the juice to lower the glycemic index of the juice.)

FATS AND OILS

While being overweight has been strongly linked with cancer risk, the overall discussion around the consumption of fats has been a bit confusing. Many act as if all fats are equal and thus suggest finding diets that reduce calories from 32.7 percent of our diets (the American average) to as low as 10 to 15 percent. Keeping fat intake low has been proven to reduce cancer risk, as cultures with the lowest fat consumption also have the lowest incidence of cancer, but studies are now suggesting that reducing fats from meats, processed oils, and dairy products is better than simply reducing calories from any kinds of fats.

How do you recognize bad fats? First, avoid all trans, hydrogenated, or partially hydrogenated fats. These are the most toxic fats and are very imflammatory. Second, avoid all deep-fried foods, which are also very inlammatory. Other bad fats include *saturated* and excessive *polyunsaturated* fats, which Americans are guilty of consuming. Since bad fats are associated with many different kinds of cancer, learn to recognize these dangerous kinds of fats and limit or avoid them. Polyunsaturated fats are typically omega-6 fats and reside primarily in most plant oils, including safflower oil, cottonseed oil, sunflower oil, soybean oil, corn oil, most salad dressings, and many processed foods and fast foods. Saturated fats come from animal products such as whole milk, marbled red meat, pork, skins of chicken and turkey, bacon, luncheon meats, cheese, ice cream, and butter. Stay away from them as much as possible.

The most dangerous fats are trans fats or hydrogenated and partly hydrogenated oils, which are heated in the presence of hydrogen and metal catalysts to increase their shelf life. This process creates *trans fats*, which are being shown in study after study as the most dangerous type of fat. While this has encouraged people to look for "no trans fats" or "trans fat free" on labels, this can be misleading, because all manufacturers have to do to get this classification is to reduce the trans fats per serving to under half a gram. While hardly anyone would call five tortilla chips, for example, a serving, if designating five tortilla chips as a serving is what is needed to get the serving of trans fats under half a gram, then that may have been done to get "no trans fats" added on the front of the bag or on the label. Marketers are very shrewd, and you must read the ingredients and avoid it if it contains hydrogenated or partially hydrogenated fat in the ingredient list. Trans fats will displace essential fatty acids in the body, but with none of their benefits, and will trigger inflammation in the body. Foods such as margarine, many types of french fries, doughnuts, pastries, and cake icing are high in trans fats.

SMOKED, PROCESSED, SALTED, OR GRILLED?

As we discussed earlier in this book, meats cooked at high temperatures produce toxic chemicals such as HCAs that would not otherwise be in meats, some of which have been linked to stomach and digestive system cancers. Smoked and processed meats should also be avoided, as well as salt-preserved foods.

Processed and fried foods (in particular meats like bacon, sausage, ham, bologna, spam, pepperoni, and salami) are typically high in *advanced glycation end products* (AGEs), which increase systemic inflammation and inhibit the immune system, which sets the stage for cancer to occur. AGEs appear in abundance in foods that are heated, pasteurized, dried, smoked, fried, or grilled. AGEs oxidize whatever they can connect with, causing the oxidative stress that is closely linked to inflammation. As such, AGEs appear to increase the risks of heart disease, diabetes, kidney disease, cancer, and other chronic conditions.

How's Your pH?

Realize that cancer thrives in an acidic body; therefore we must learn how to alkalinize our tissues. Alkalizing foods and beverages help raise the pH of your tissues, which enables your body to expel more toxins and usually slows the growth of tumors. Acidic foods reverse this process and thus encourage the retention of toxins that can lead to cell damage and mutations and the growth of tumors.[4]

The place to start with this is to make sure you have a good, supply of clean, alkaline water in your home and where you work, even if you have to bring it with you every day yourself. I like to say that water is the ultimate detoxifier. Clean, alkaline water without any impurities unburdens your liver and kidneys and helps your colon function as it should. It also helps to raise the pH of your tissues, encouraging detoxification on the cellular level.

If we don't detoxify regularly, toxins can build up in our bodies, causing inflammation, stressing our liver, and damaging our DNA, the molecular building blocks of life, causing originally healthy cells to mutate and start the cancer process. City air is one of the biggest offenders. Hydrocarbons, smog, cigarette smoke, and other toxic substances often contaminate it.

In rural areas, pesticides, many of which are carcinogenic, are sprayed on American crops each year. Tons and tons of poisonous garbage sits rotting in toxic waste sites, and many of these sites in America threaten to seep their toxins into the water supply. Our farm animals feed on antibiotics and hormones as well. As cancer-causing agents increase all around us, we must follow God-given strategies to win the war against their harmful effects.

Because of the concern these pose, I encourage my patients to use pH strips to test their urine, especially first thing in the morning and during the day if needed. Generally my patients have a pH of 5.0, which is about a hundred times more acidic that it should be. A pH of 7.0 is considered neutral; above that is considered alkaline. A healthy urine pH is slightly alkaline, between 7.0 and 7.5. (Note that a highly alkaline pH can make your body more susceptible to infection, so again, slightly alkaline is a proper balance.)

To reverse a high-acidity level, I suggest you drink fresh, juiced organic vegetables with breakfast and in the midafternoon. Adding 1 or 2 tablespoons of pulp back into the juices will also help lower the glycemic index of the juice. Add lemon or lime to your water throughout the day. Phytonutrient-rich powders such as Green Superfood mixed into juices or smoothies also help cleanse and alkalize the body. A great source for juicing recipes is Gwynn Palmer's *Eat Well and Live!* and my book *Toxic Relief.*

Juices made with sprouts, wheatgrass, barley grass, oat grass, spirulina, chlorella, and blue-green algae are wonderful for reversing acidity, plus they are extremely high in chlorophyll. Chlorophyll has been found to have anticancer effects, since it protects the DNA from damaging radiation. These foods have also been shown to have antiviral, antitumor, and anti-inflammatory properties. In effect, such foods can actually inhibit carcinogens in cooked meats and even in cigarette smoke. I recommend that patients make a chlorophyll drink containing one or more of these potent power foods on a regular basis. Warning: if you have a high serum iron or ferritin level, you may need to limit your green foods. (See Appendix A.)

To keep your body's pH balanced, you should eat one serving of vegetables and one fruit (or another alkalizing food) for every acidic food you eat (every meat or grain). By and large, alkalizing foods are also anti-inflammatory foods, and acidic foods are typically inflammatory, so following the dictates of the Mediterranean diet with an anti-inflammatory twist is already a great place to have addressed this. While I do not really have the space in this book to list all of the alkalizing and acidifying foods here, I do have a detailed description of them in my books *The Seven Pillars of Health*, *Toxic Relief* and *Get Healthy Through Detox and Fasting*, which I would encourage you to read in determining your overall cancer- and disease-defeating meal plans. (See Appendix B.)

Furthermore, there is growing evidence that tumors do not do as well in an alkaline environment. Italian oncologist Dr. Tullio Simoncini has even been experimenting with treating tumors with sodium bicarbonate, common baking soda, and has had some remarkable results. In his remarkable thesis *Cancer Is a Fungus*, Dr. Simoncini presents his case for applying baking soda directly to cancerous areas and explains that it destroys the fungal colonies lying at the heart of the tumors and thus dissolves the cancer. The treatment seems to work best for cancers of the throat, colon, intestines, rectal area, and digestive tract, according to Dr. Simoncini, since they are easier to reach by ingesting baking soda.[5] While this treatment is still under investigation, I would strong recommend that you start alkalinizing your urine by drinking alkaline water, juicing, adding lemon and lime to your water, and taking supplements high in chlorophyll. Also, aluminum-free baking soda from the health food store or Vaxa Buffered pH are excellent supplements to raise the urine pH. (See Appendix A.) Do not use aluminum-free baking soda if you have hypertension.

THREATENING THE THREATS

The "threats" we've been looking at in this chapter are not the last word on our health. As Christians, we have the Lord at our side, making sure that nothing brings us ultimate defeat—not even death itself. Here is how the apostle Paul put it:

> If God is for us, who can ever be against us? Since he did not spare even his own Son but gave him up for us all, won't he also give us everything else?
> —ROMANS 8:31–32

However, faith works by the promises of God and adhering to His wisdom. Choosing the right things to eat that God naturally gave us in Creation to replace the wrong things, we can have all that much more confidence that His promises of divine health are ours. Continue to build your faith and your wisdom to defeat cancer as you continue to explore *The New Bible Cure for Cancer.*

A **BIBLE CURE** Prayer for You

*Dear God, I believe in Your promises. Please
help build my faith in the following ways:*

_____

_____

_____

Thank You, in the name of Jesus Christ, the great Healer! Amen.

A **BIBLE CURE** Prescription
Strengthening Your Faith
to Beat Cancer

Take a moment to consider your level of faith in God's promises as it
relates to your battle against cancer. As you do, think about things you
can do to continue to build your faith and wisdom about how to live
in the health God planned for us all when He first created the earth.

Chapter 5

NUTRIENTS THAT GIVE YOU
THAT EXTRA ADVANTAGE

WHILE WE HAVE already discussed the key "power foods" that can give our bodies tremendous defenses against cancer, we now need to go to the next level and see what supplements we can add to those to make sure we are getting what we need every day. It can be hard to plan your daily meals to include every food you should eat to get the maximum anticancer benefits, but by adding a daily supplement regimen of phytonutrients, supplements that boost the immune system, and anticancer nutrients, you can have a great deal of protection from their benefits alone. These are often called *phytonutrients*. They have existed in our foods since God first created the earth, and science is just beginning to discover their incredible potential.

A **BIBLE CURE** *Health Fact*

The Power Given to Us in Plants

Phytochemicals (*phyto-* being a Greek prefix for "plant") are the new nutritional frontier, and already research on them has speeded into fast-forward. At a time when more and more cancers are tagged as diet related, the National Cancer Institute is so convinced of the potential of phytochemicals that it has committed millions of dollars for research. Tens of thousands of phytochemicals exist in the foods we eat—nearly all of them in fruits and vegetables.[1] Working together, these "plant nutrients" show incredible potential for reducing inflammation, inhibiting tumor growth, blocking carcinogenic toxins, and increasing the number of natural killer cells roaming our bodies looking for cellular rebels.

> Fruit trees of all kinds will grow along both sides of the river.... The fruit will be for food and the leaves for healing.
>
> —EZEKIEL 47:12

Exciting, isn't it? You probably want to know more about the phytonutrients and supplements you need to live healthy and fight disease and how to get them into your daily diet. Well, here's the info you need! (These are presented in no special order.)

COMPREHENSIVE MULTIVITAMINS
(WITH MINERALS)

Every good health-promoting supplement routine should start with a comprehensive multivitamin and mineral. While I have gone into a brief description of individual vitamins, minerals, and nutrients in the following pages, it is important to remember that fighting cancer starts with being healthy and maintaining a healthy, strong immune system. Research shows that from a young age, your body handles fifty to one hundred mutated—i.e., potentially cancerous—cells almost every day of your life, but it is only as your body and its systems get stressed with age, lack of sleep, being overweight, not getting enough exercise, poor diet, smoking, too much stress from work or life, an excessive toxic burden, and compromised liver function that cancer can get a foothold in your body. I strongly recommend *The Seven Pillars of Health* to learn more about these issues. Staying at a healthy weight, getting adequate rest, coping with stress, exercising regularly, eating right, and getting the proper daily recommended allowances of the correct nutrients is the best plan for keeping cancer out of your life or decreasing its potency as you fight to eliminate it.

So find a good quality, comprehensive daily multivitamin with minerals to use as the basis of your supplement routine. I discuss this in detail in my book *The Seven Pillars of Health*. Many multivitamins are divided by sex or according to health concerns, so make sure to add to those the individual supplements that are needed for your particular concerns or health issues.

The Food and Nutrition Board of the Institute of Medicine has replaced the old RDA (recommended daily allowance) with

DRI (dietary reference intake) values. Some of the nutrient levels in the DRI are higher than in the RDA. A good multi-vitamin should include the following vitamins and minerals for the prevention of cancer:

- **Folic acid:** We need the eight B vitamins on a daily basis. However, perhaps the most important B vitamin for cancer prevention is folic acid. Just a mild folic acid deficiency may promote cervical dysplasia, a premalignant condition. Folic acid is important for DNA repair. In one study, patients taking the highest amount of folic acid had a significant reduction in the risk of developing premalignant polyps of the colon.[2]

- **Vitamin A:** This vitamin inhibits the development of cancerous tumors and can promote remission of premalignant oral lesions termed leukoplakia. The four fat-soluble vitamins A, D, E, and K, may be depleted in cancer patients due to fat malabsorption, which is so common, especially in advanced cancers.

- **Zinc:** Inadequate levels of zinc affect natural killer cell and T-cell activity, which decreases the immune system's ability to defend your body. Low levels of zinc also slow wound healing from surgery and tissue repair from chemotherapy and radiation. Zinc also needs to be balanced with copper.

- **Copper:** This mineral is also very important for the healthy function of the immune system. Copper deficiency is associated with decreased natural killer cell activity.

- **Chromium:** This mineral works with insulin to stabilize the blood sugar levels, which turns down the fuel supply for cancer. Remember, cancer's favorite fuel is sugar.

SELENIUM

Selenium and sulfur are part of glutathione peroxidase, the body's most important antioxidant and detoxifying agent. Animal studies have shown that selenium helps inhibit the formation of tumors and also may slow their growth.

Selenium is a very important mineral for our bodies, yet most Americans only get between 60 and 100 mcg of it a day instead of the recommended 200 mcg.[3] This mineral helps to prevent damaged DNA molecules from replicating and repeating the mistakes that become cell mutations. More than one hundred studies have been done with animals and have shown selenium to be a powerful preventative of tumor formations. In human trials it has also been shown as a strong preventative as well as slowing existing cancers, particularly prostate cancer. In one study it cut the incidence of lung cancer by nearly 50 percent.[4] While research continues on this valuable mineral, it is not too early to make sure you are getting the daily recommend amount of it in your multivitamin. I recommend 200 mcg a day of selenium.

Vitamin D₃

Is it possible that sunlight could be a preventative to cancer? Recent research seems to indicate that higher levels of vitamin D, which the skin will manufacture in our bodies when exposed to sunlight, may reduce the risk of breast, prostate, and other cancers by as much as 66 percent.

In one study done with 1,760 nurses, study coauthor Cedric Garland said:

> The data is very clear, showing that individuals in the group with the lowest blood levels had the highest rates of breast cancer, and the breast cancer rates dropped as the blood levels of 25-hydroxyvitamin D increased.... The serum level associated with a 50 percent reduction in risk could be maintained by taking 2,000 international units of vitamin D_3 daily, plus, when the weather permits, spending 10 to 15 minutes a day in the sun.[5]

JoEllen Welsh, research of State University of New York at Albany, has been conducting research on vitamin D for twenty-five years. She found that when mice injected with breast cancer cells were treated with vitamin D, after several weeks the tumors shrank by 50 percent, and some even disappeared.[6]

Of a study published in the *American Journal of Preventative Medicine* in 2007, study coauthor Edward Gorham said:

> Through this meta-analysis we found that raising the serum level of 25-hydroxyvitamin D to 34 ng/ml would reduce the incidence of colorectal cancer

by half.... We project a two-thirds reduction in incidence with serum levels of 46 ng/ml, which corresponds to a daily intake of 2,000 IU of vitamin D_3. This would be best achieved with a combination of diet, supplements and 10 to 15 minutes per day in the sun.[7]

I would advocate following their advice and adding 2,000 to 5,000 IU of vitamin D_3 to your daily supplements. I also check 250HD3 serum levels and adjust the patient's dose of vitamin D_3 until I reach a level of 50 to 100 ng/ml. The patient with low levels of vitamin D_3 may need to take 5,000 units of vitamin D_3 a day for three to four months and then have their vitamin D_3 level rechecked. Most patients can eventually be maintained on a dose of 2,000 to 4,000 IU a day. (See Appendix A.)

RESVERATROL

As we already discussed in chapter 3, resveratrol, a compound found in red grapes and red wine, has wonderful anticarcinogenic effects—and is available without the alcohol in supplements. (See Appendix A.) Resveratrol has the ability to interfere with several processes that are important in the progression of tumors and is very effective in preventing breast, colon, and esophageal cancer.

OMEGA-3 FATTY ACIDS (EFA AND DHA)

A higher intake of omega-3 fatty acids, obtained through eating cold-water fish such as salmon and sardines, or more conveniently through taking pharmaceutical grade fish oil capsules, has been linked with lower inflammation and lower cancer risk, as well as a multitude of other health benefits. There is good evidence that these fatty acids repair cells and DNA, keeping mutations from being made in cellular reproduction. They work to "switch off" production of molecules necessary to the cancer cycle and "switch on" genes that signal for apoptosis (cell death) in cells before they can become full-blown tumors.

Due to these positive effects, I encourage taking a daily pharmaceutical fish oil supplement that is not rancid. A good dosage for most people to include with their normal supplements would be 300 mg three times a day, with 180 mg EPA and 120 mg DHA contained in each capsule.

CURCUMIN

Curcumin, the valuable compound found in the spice turmeric, may help to prevent or fight prostate, pancreatic, breast, and colon cancers. It probably does this because curcumin inhibits the COX-2 enzyme that promotes inflammation. Aspirin also inhibits the COX-2 enzyme and helps prevent colon cancer. Curcumin can also be taken in supplement form. Remember that it is an antioxidant several times more powerful than vitamin E and that piperine, a compound found in pepper, increases its absorption. Because of this and the incredible health benefits of curcumin for multiple diseases, I suggest you have 600 to 1200 mg of turmeric once or twice a day in a supplement that also includes piperine to increase its effectiveness.

MELATONIN

Melatonin has long been touted as a natural sleep aid, but did you know it also has significant anticancer benefits? Melatonin has been shown to improve immune system function, help individuals cope with stress, and diminish certain aspects of aging, as well as help fight fibrocystic breast diseases and breast and colon cancers. It also demonstrates protection against the toxic side effects of chemotherapy and radiation therapy and improves healing after cancer surgery.[8] Those who already sleep well may not need a melatonin supplement to help their natural production of it. For information on melatonin, please refer to *The New Bible Cure for Sleep Disorders.* I usually recommend 1 to 6 mg of melatonin dissolved in the mouth at bedtime or if you awaken during the night. (See Appendix A.)

INOSITOL HEXAPHOSPHATE (IP6)

Inositol hexaphosphate (IP6) has strong antioxidant and antitumor functions. It may be able to cause cancer cells to mature and eventually go on to die in a normal cell cycle. IP6 also strengthens our immunity and boosts the activity and number of our natural killer (NK) cells. This powerful antioxidant also comes from whole-grain cereals, legumes, and soybean seeds. It resides in the bran layer of rice and wheat seeds. In corn, it is found in the germ portion of the kernel.

Researchers at the University of Colorado Cancer Center found that two genes activated by IP6 play a pivotal role in halting tumor growth and promoting apoptosis in prostate cancer cells.[9] Another study has shown that tumor regression took place in people who took 8 grams of IP6 for three to four weeks, which would be roughly the amount found in 12 ounces of whole corn kernels. Another benefit is that it binds to certain metals to help detoxify our bodies.

> And you know that God anointed Jesus of Nazareth with the Holy Spirit and with power. Then Jesus went around doing good and healing all who were oppressed by the devil, for God was with him.
>
> —ACTS 10:38

IP6 is found naturally in all of our cells, but when found in food it is bound to proteins and must be separated from them for the body to absorb. However, the enzyme that does this will also commonly damage it, making it difficult to use in our bodies. This is not a problem when taken in a pure form, so it can be wonderfully beneficial as a supplement. I usually recommend 3.2 g of IP6 powder (one scoop) taken two times daily—one to be taken in the morning and one in the evening.

DIINDOLYLMETHANE (DIM) AND INDOLE-3-CARBINOL (I3C)

Indole-3-carbinol (I3C), one of the powerful compounds found in cruciferous vegetable that the body turns into valuable diindolylmethane (DIM), can also be taken in supplement form. DIM is the most active cruciferous substance for promoting estrogen metabolism. While this does not change the value of your grandmother's advice to "Eat your broccoli, cauliflower, and brussels sprouts!" it can still help you get some of their most effective benefits without struggling to chew them up and swallow them. These compounds seem especially beneficial for those at risk of the hormone-driven cancers of the breasts, prostate, and cervix. Because it modulates estrogen, pregnant women should avoid these supplements, but for others concerned with hormone-driven cancers, you should take a daily supplement of cruciferous vegetable extracts. I usually recommend 100 mg of DIM two times a day and/or 120 mg of IC3 twice a day. DIM is more stable than IC3, so it is more preferable.

CALCIUM D-GLUCARATE

Calcium D-glucarate is a natural detoxifier and supports the body's detox systems. It is extracted from fruits such as apples, oranges, and grapefruit and from cruciferous vegetables such as broccoli and brussels sprouts.

In order to eliminate certain toxins and hormones from our bodies, glucuronic acid is attached to them in the liver and then excreted in the bile. D-glucarate inhibits beta-glucuronidase, which is a bacterial enzyme that promotes hormone-driven cancers such as breast, prostate, and colon cancers. It may also reduce the risk of lung, liver, skin, and other types of cancers. I recommend a supplement including 200 mg of calcium D-glucarate a day with or without food. (See Appendix A.)

> He send his word and healed them, snatching them from the door of death.
>
> —PSALM 107:20

GLUTATHIONE

Glutathione is the most important antioxidant in the body. It also functions as a detoxifier of the body, neutralizing toxins and heavy metals as well as quenching free radicals. The reduced form of glutathione is the active form and is abbreviated as GSH. Glutathione is water soluble and concentrated mainly in the blood and cytoplasm portion of every cell in your body. The liver has the highest per cell concentration of glutathione.

Glutathione-promoting supplements actually decrease glutathione in cancer cells and increase GSH levels in immune cells. This helps to fuel the immune system to both prevent and fight cancer as it makes cancer cells more susceptible to any type of therapy.

Also, vitamin D_3, according to scientific literature, decreases levels of glutathione and increases production of free radicals in every type of cancer cell. In other words, one way vitamin D_3 protects us against cancer is by robbing the cancer cell of glutathione, which usually protects the cancer cell from destruction.

I recommend glutathione-promoting supplements to every patient with cancer or everyone who wants to prevent cancer. (See Appendix A.) If you desire more information on nutritional supplements and antioxidants, please refer to *The Seven Pillars of Health*.

THE POWER OF ENZYMES

Though his theories are still largely controversial, the story of dentist William Kelley is a testimony to the power of diet, nutrients, enzymes, and detoxification in the treatment and prevention of cancer. Dr. Kelley was diagnosed with inoperable pancreatic cancer in 1967 and was told he only had months to live. In response, he began experimenting with the regimen of a natural foods diet, proper supplements, high-dose enzyme therapy, and a detox program that cleansed him of toxins. This cured him of the deadly cancer he faced. Not only that, but also he lived on until the age of seventy-nine, finally passing away in 2005, roughly thirty-eight years after his diagnosis. Kelley's method also worked for thousands of others over that time. His book, *One Answer to Cancer*, is still widely referenced today. His theories were based on the work of Dr. John Beard, who published *The Enzyme Theory of Cancer* in 1911.

Kelley believed that cancer was a pancreatic-enzyme deficiency caused by the body being overloaded with secondhand proteins (from the meats we eat), and thus the enzymes were not able to digest the foreign proteins known as cancer. There are twenty-two different types of enzymes produced in the body, most of them by the pancreas. This production is one of the things that wane as we grow older. Chronic enzyme deficiency weakens the immune system. It is possible to replace such enzymes through the foods we eat and by taking proteolytic and digestive enzyme supplements.

Cancer cells, like nearly all pathogens, are enclosed in fibrin, a protein-based coating that makes it difficult for the immune system to recognize. It is fifteen times thicker than the membranes of normal cells. When there are enough of these digestive enzymes floating around in our systems, they will eat through that thick cell membrane and expose cancer to the arresting power of the immune system; when enzymes are not there, cancers can go undetected and undeterred.

Dr. Nicholas Gonzalez studied Kelley's research and patients as a medical school student and is one of the main proponents of enzyme therapy today. His tests with it, however, have yet to live up to the results in Kelley's life and in the lives of some of his patients; thus what has come to be known as "the Kelley

Protocol" is still largely under debate. There are still nutritionists, naturopaths, and other nutritional doctors who monitor patients on the Kelley Protocol in managing cancer. I do not recommend this program unless you are being followed by a doctor trained in the Kelley Protocol.

Regardless, I believe proteolytic enzyme therapy and the Kelley Protocol is still worth considering, especially what Kelley believed about the foods we eat and keeping our bodies detoxified. If you are facing cancer, it would certainly be worth looking further into the research and discussing enzyme therapy with a nutritional doctor. Smaller doses of digestive enzymes may also have health benefits for those looking at them as a preventative supplement to be taken with meals.

ADVICE THAT HAS WITHSTOOD THE TEST OF TIME

Long ago, God told the people of Israel:

> If you will listen carefully to the voice of the LORD your God and do what is right in his sight, obeying his commands and keeping all his decrees, then I will not make you suffer any of the diseases I sent on the Egyptians; for I am the LORD who heals you.
> —EXODUS 15:26

This promise is for us too. He is still the Lord who heals us today, and I believe He still calls us to listen carefully to His voice and to do what is right. That must be our approach when it comes to all aspects of living, including how we act, what we eat, and the supplements from His creation that we add to our daily diets. The original Patent Holder in the universe still knows what is best for His creation. It has just taken humanity time to understand it and to begin to undo the bad habits we have fallen into as we got away from God's wisdom. There is no question that God's ways are still above our ways, even when it comes to what we eat!

A BIBLE CURE Prayer for You

Father, I thank You for all of the wonderful vitamins, minerals, and nutrients that You put into this earth and its plants in Your plan to give me a long and healthy life. Give me the wisdom to understand their importance and the daily discipline to take them as I should. Multiply their benefits in me to give me the abundance of life You promised through Your Son, Jesus Christ.

I thank You in His name, the name above every name, Jesus. Amen.

A **Bible Cure** Prescription

Assembling Your Nutritional Weapons Against Cancer

With what you have learned so far, now you should be ready to load up your "daily supplement routine" arsenal against cancer with powerful vitamins, minerals, and nutrients. Evaluate how well you are doing now, and determine to increase your intake of these valuable food extracts in the coming weeks. Put an *x* on the line where you are now and ✓ on the line for what you want to do in the days ahead.

Take a daily multivitamin:

1 ___ 2 ___ 3 ___ 4 ___ 5 ___ 6 ___ 7 ___
Never   Sometimes   Often

Get your daily vitamin D_3 (2,000–5,000 IU a day):

1 ___ 2 ___ 3 ___ 4 ___ 5 ___ 6 ___ 7 ___
Never   Sometimes   Often

Take a resveratrol supplement:

1 ___ 2 ___ 3 ___ 4 ___ 5 ___ 6 ___ 7 ___
Never   Sometimes   Often

Take pharmaceutical-grade fish oil capsules daily:

1 ___ 2 ___ 3 ___ 4 ___ 5 ___ 6 ___ 7 ___
Never   Sometimes   Often

Take a curcumin supplement:

1 ___ 2 ___ 3 ___ 4 ___ 5 ___ 6 ___ 7 ___
Never   Sometimes   Often

Take melatonin before bedtime and before chemotherapy and radiation:

1 ___ 2 ___ 3 ___ 4 ___ 5 ___ 6 ___ 7 ___
Never   Sometimes   Often

Take IP6:

1 ___ 2 ___ 3 ___ 4 ___ 5 ___ 6 ___ 7 ___
Never   Sometimes   Often

Take DIM and/or I3C (cruciferous veggie):

1 ___ 2 ___ 3 ___ 4 ___ 5 ___ 6 ___ 7 ___
Never   Sometimes   Often

Take a calcium D-glucarate supplement:

1 ___ 2 ___ 3 ___ 4 ___ 5 ___ 6 ___ 7 ___
Never   Sometimes   Often

Take 200 mcg of selenium daily:

1 ___ 2 ___ 3 ___ 4 ___ 5 ___ 6 ___ 7 ___
Never   Sometimes   Often

Take a glutathione-promoting supplement:

1 ___ 2 ___ 3 ___ 4 ___ 5 ___ 6 ___ 7 ___
Never   Sometimes   Often

Take omega-3 fats:

1 ___ 2 ___ 3 ___ 4 ___ 5 ___ 6 ___ 7 ___
Never   Sometimes   Often

Take digestive enzymes with meals:

1 ___ 2 ___ 3 ___ 4 ___ 5 ___ 6 ___ 7 ___
Never   Sometimes   Often

Resveratrol, vitamin D_3, curcumin, melatonin, DIM, calcium D-glucarate, omega-3 fats, selenium, and glutathione-boosting supplements are for prevention of cancer. If you have cancer, take the above and add IP6.

Chapter 6

THE CANCER-BEATING LIFESTYLE

G OD'S WILL FOR the people of the earth was readily demonstrated in everything Jesus said and did:

> Jesus traveled throughout the region of Galilee, teaching in the synagogues and announcing the Good News about the Kingdom. And he healed every kind of disease and illness.
> —MATTHEW 4:23

You don't find a lot of admonitions in the Bible for people to exercise, do you? Of course not! And why? Because people walked or rode horses or donkeys everywhere. They didn't need more exercise because their daily lives were filled with it working their farms, carrying their wares to market, walking across town to meet friends or family, or working in their shops as things were made by hand. Even cooking started with going out to get the wood to build the fire. People in Jesus's day had exercise built into their lives, and it was a health benefit He never had to mention. I strongly recommend my book *Get Fit and Live!* for exercises to prevent cancer. Rebounding is especially important for lymphatic drainage, which removes cellular waste and toxins.

In the same way, there are other lifestyle modifications we can make outside of controlling what we eat that will help us keep cancer out of our lives. It is worth taking another look at those here in the following pages before we leave our discussion of *The New Bible Cure for Cancer*.

QUIT SMOKING

The most important lifestyle modification in preventing cancer—and a handful of other deadly diseases for that matter—is to get away from the air pollution of smoking. If you're a smoker, it's time to stop smoking! Secondly, whether you smoke or not, avoid secondhand smoke. Cigarette smoke fills the air with over four thousand different chemicals, fifty of which have been proven to be cancer-causing.[1] Further, these chemicals trigger significant free-radical reactions, the very cell-damaging work that mutates cells in the first place and makes them susceptible to carcinogenesis.

The bottom line is that smoking and even inhaling secondhand smoke accelerates aging, causes tremendous free-radical damage, introduces hundreds of toxins into the body, and sets the stage for cancer. It is imperative that you take steps today to get cigarette smoke out of your life for good, starting from this very moment.

REDUCE OR ELIMINATE ALCOHOL CONSUMPTION

Alcohol consumption has been repeatedly linked to several different cancers, particularly mouth, esophageal, laryngeal, pharyngeal, breast, and liver cancers. According to the American Cancer Society, "The more someone drinks, the higher his or her risk of developing some kinds of cancer. Reducing the amount of alcohol a person drinks will sharply reduce cancer risk."[2]

If you do choose to drink alcohol, do so only in moderation, which means two drinks or less for men and one or less for women a day. (A drink is one 12-ounce beer, 4 ounces of wine, 1.5 ounces of 80-proof spirits, or 1 ounce of 100-proof spirits.) I also suggest only drinking with meals. Personally, I do not recommend drinking any alcohol at all since too many people find it difficult to stop after only one or two glasses. In that light, one capsule of Living Resveratrol has the health benefits of six hundred glasses of red wine with no toxic effects. So, if you choose not to drink, as I do, Living Resveratrol—or some other resveratrol supplement—will give you all of the benefits of red wine without the drawbacks of its alcohol content.

YOUR HEALTHY WEIGHT IS YOUR STRONGEST ALLY

While researchers are still working out the kinks of many of the suggestions and studies quoted in this book, all of them do seem to agree on at least one point—the Western world is killing itself slowly by choosing to be obese and far too sedentary. As part of the 2009 American Association of Cancer Research 100th Annual Meeting, Harvard School of Public Medicine nutritionist Walter Willet presented an overview entitled "Diet, Nutrition and Cancer: The Search for Truth." In it he said:

> The estimate that diet contributes to around 30 to 35 percent of cancers is still reasonable, but much of this is related to being overweight and inactive. At this point, being overweight is second only to smoking

as a clear and avoidable cause of cancer.... People should stay as lean as they can.[3]

Your body mass index (BMI) should be between 18.5 and 24.9 as a healthy weight for an adult. If you are overweight or obese according to the BMI, change your diet and read my book *Dr. Colbert's "I Can Do This" Diet*. Also find an exercise routine you can stick with and read my book *Get Fit and Live!* Getting down to your healthy weight is one of the best things you can do for your body to prevent cancer. Belly fat raises the CRP (C-reactive protein), and elevated CRP is associated with an increased risk of cancer.

EXERCISE DAILY

How often do you exercise during the week? Did you know that getting out and jogging, walking, or bicycling—or participating in any type of regular, moderate form of exertion—can help you avoid cancer? It's time to get up off that couch and get active! Regular exercise is one of the best ways to maintain good health. Besides, I have a feeling that God takes pleasure in the health of our bodies:

> He gives power to the weak and strength to the powerless.... Those who trust in the Lord will find new strength. They will soar high on wings like eagles. They will run and not grow weary. They will walk and not faint.
>
> —ISAIAH 40:29, 31

Numerous studies have shown that people who exercise regularly have lower incidences of cancer in general. Another great thing about exercise is that it makes our digested food move more quickly through the GI tract. That way it can't sit there and produce potentially cancer-causing toxins. Exercise also lowers the risks of endometrial and breast cancers by reducing a woman's body fat (which produces estrogen, an encourager of several cancers).

> He forgives all my sins and heals all my diseases.
> —PSALM 103:3

The best form of exercise is aerobic exercise, which includes brisk walking, cycling, rebounding, swimming, or jogging. Some doctors say that just thirty minutes of exercise every other day can reduce the risk of breast cancer by 75 percent! You see, cancer cells are anaerobic, which means they don't thrive in high-oxygen environments. Exercise pumps oxygen to your cells, giving your body an added ability to win the war against cancer. I encourage you to read *Get Fit and Live!* which includes an entire chapter of exercise workouts for people battling cancer.

SLEEP IS A REWARD OF RIGHTEOUSNESS— AND GOOD FOR YOUR IMMUNE SYSTEM!

Research suggests that inadequate sleep and rest may shorten your life by eight to ten years, if not more, because you have weakened your immune function and probably decreased your natural killer cell count, which is your first line of defense against cancer.

A lot of people think of sleep as a time when everything shuts down, but the truth is your body does a lot of important repair work and immune surveillance while you are asleep. Lack of sleep may also raise cortisol levels, which suppress immune function. Melatonin, a compound we discussed in the last chapter, has anticarcinogenic properties and is produced while you sleep, so cutting sleep short over and over again is often what leads to being deficient in it. No wonder the Bible tells us:

> It is useless for you to work so hard from early morning until late at night, anxiously working for food to eat; for God gives rest to his loved ones.
>
> —PSALM 127:2

All of us need at least seven to nine hours of sleep a night (eight hours is usually ideal), and if you are not getting that, you are not giving your body the time it needs *daily* to repair and rejuvenate itself. If you are suffering from insomnia, you are weakening your immune system and increasing your risk of cancer. For more information on insomnia, refer to my book *The New Bible Cure for Sleep Disorders*.

DEDICATE YOUR DAYS TO GOD

I want to remind you to keep praying and seeking God as you make these dietary and lifestyle changes! Take a lesson from the prophet:

> As my life was slipping away, I remembered the LORD, and my earnest prayer went out to you.
>
> —JONAH 2:7

Even if you don't feel like praying, keep on approaching the throne of grace every day; your prayers do come before the Lord as much as your daily decisions and behavior do. I know it can be difficult. If you have some form of cancer, the pain and weakness can bring on bouts of discouragement. But those who wrote the Bible learned about God in the same ways that you and I learn about Him. They became discouraged and fearful at times too, so David wrote these words of truth and encouragement:

> The LORD hears his people when they call to him for help. He rescues them from all their troubles. The LORD is close to the brokenhearted; he rescues those whose spirits are crushed. The righteous person faces many troubles, but the LORD comes to the rescue each time.
> —PSALM 34:17–19

These are certainly words to live by.

A **BIBLE CURE** Prayer for You

Father, guide my days and my steps as I seek to follow You with all of my heart. Keep me free of sickness and disease, especially any form of cancer that would try to keep me from fulfilling all You have called me to do on this earth. Guide me to walk in divine health and in ways that prevent disease so it is never an issue. Heal my mind and attitudes as much as my body, and make me an example of all I should be as Your follower.

As I love You with all my strength, heart, soul, and mind, strengthen each of those areas through the power of Your Spirit.

I ask this in the name above every name, Jesus Christ, my Lord and Savior. Amen.

A **BIBLE CURE** Prescription

What Do You Need?

The promise of Scripture is clear when it comes to praying for what you need. This applies to all your circumstances, even when you face cancer and seek healing. Listen to the words of Jesus: "And so I tell you, keep on asking, and you will receive what you ask for. Keep on seeking, and you will find. Keep on knocking, and the door will be opened to you. For everyone who asks, receives" (Luke 11:9–10). Think about what you need most in order to apply these words to your life these days. Mark the lines below with the specific letter(s) denoting your particular need:

I = I need more INFORMATION about health and/or insight into God's will.

C = I need more COURAGE to face my enemy, cancer.

C = I need more COMMITMENT so I can be self-disciplined and make good choices.

F = I need more FAITH in order to believe God's promises and persevere in my trials.

(I Can Conquer Fear)

___ When you hear about new treatments, medicines, and therapies

___ When your doctor says you need chemotherapy

___ When you feel impatient with God's timing

___ When you've experienced another health setback

___ When you're depressed because of the stress and pain of cancer

___ When you must relocate to a new place for health reasons

___ When you worry that you might get sick (or sicker)

___ When you can't eat the things you want

___ When you have to make lifestyle changes because of sickness

___ Other: _____

Think: What things help the most when you're discouraged in your battles? What first steps can you take right now to pursue at least one of those things?

I tell patients diagnosed with cancer to reframe how they see the diagnosis of cancer. Instead of feeling fearful, anxious, and hopeless with the diagnosis of cancer, boldly declare, "God can answer," and you are seeing cancer from God's point of view or God's perspective. No longer do you say, "I have cancer." You say, "God can answer."

Chapter 7

TAKE A SOUL CHECK—AND A WALK

S OMEONE ONCE SAID that the best way out is always through. It's true in your fight against cancer. By combining God's natural foods and nutrients with His positive prescriptions for the mind, emotions, and spirit, you can build a powerful immune system that can knock cancer to its knees. No toxin will be able to get a foothold in your body, and fear will gain no place in your mind.

The New Bible Cure for Cancer offers a bold, fearless response to meet the challenge of cancer, and that response includes faith in the powerful promises of God's living Word.

TAKE FIVE NOW

We've talked about taking various foods and supplements throughout this book. These focus on strengthening and protecting your physical body, but what do you take for the mind and spirit—two of the other parts of you that greatly affect your overall well-being? Consider these six suggestions:

1. Take refuge in the Scriptures. God's Word breaks the destructive power of certain deadly emotions, such as fear, rage, hatred, resentment, bitterness, and shame. I encourage you to quote scriptures related to them at least three times a day on a continuous basis. Also read and meditate on Bible passages like

1 Corinthians 13, the chapter on God's definition of love, since there is no greater force in the universe than the power of God's love. It is able to break the bondage of any destructive emotion.

2. Take up positive attitudes. Related to Scripture reading is the practice of putting on the positive, healthy emotions like love, joy, peace, patience, kindness, goodness, and self-control. We know that certain emotions are associated with lowered immune function. Approaching life with the biblical attitude will help you avoid the damaging effects of stress, fear, and worry. Several decades ago, S. I. McMillen, author of the best-selling *None of These Diseases*, confirmed what I'm saying:

> Peace does not come in capsules! This is regrettable because medical science recognizes that [deadly] emotions such as fear, sorrow, envy, resentment, and hatred are responsible for the majority of our sicknesses. Estimates vary from 60 percent to nearly 100 percent.[1]

3. Take time to offer a blessing. Naturally, I recommend that everyone bless their food prior to eating it. Blessing the food and then choosing to eat unhealthy foods is unlikely to protect you since Galatians 6:7 says, "God is not mocked; for whatever a man sows, that he will also reap" (NKJV). Too many Christians are blessing toxic foods on a regular basis. Lay the sugars, high-glycemic foods, and fried foods on the altar, and choose life more abundant by eating more living foods. We all slip up at times, and because of that we need to constantly remember to rely on God's strength and wisdom more than anything else.

Simply forgive yourself for slipping and affirm your commitment to following a healthy diet.

4. Practice forgiveness and gratitude. After losing his son Dirk in a tragic accident, German oncologist Ryke Geerd Hamer developed testicular carcinoma. The connection between loss and illness inspired him to conduct extensive research on thousands of cancer patients, concluding that all had suffered some shock or trauma before their illness. Hamer's research showed that a severe shock or trauma causes a focus of activity in the brain called an HH (Hamerschenherd), which appears as concentric rings centered on a precise point of the brain on a CT scan. As soon as the HH appears, the organ controlled by that part of the brain registers a functional transformation (a growth, tissue loss, or loss of function). If the trauma is resolved, according to Hamer, the cancerous or necrotic process is reversed to repair damage and return the patient to health.

In my practice I address the traumas from patients' pasts as well as leading them through what I call "Forgiveness Therapy" as part of their treatment. I discuss the connections between emotions and the body in several of my books, including the attitude of gratitude, which takes your eyes off of whatever circumstances you may be facing and puts them on the Deliverer from bad circumstances and the Healer of diseases. I recommend you start each day by identifying at least twenty or thirty specific things, both big and small, for which you are grateful. You can do this with your family at the breakfast table or alone as you get ready for your day. When you do, it sets the tone for your daily conversations and thoughts that will keep you mindful of how wonderful life really is walking in the path ordered for you by God. Stress really can't get a hold on you if you do this every day.

5. *Take a laughter break.* Some of us hardly ever laugh, especially patients with cancer. Some haven't laughed in years, but we need to do so often. In fact, one of the best ways to prevent cancer is to laugh. The Book of Proverbs says, "A cheerful heart is good medicine, but a broken spirit saps a person's strength" (Prov. 17:22). Excessive stress is quite dangerous because it increases our cortisol levels, which then typically suppresses the immune system. I recommend ten belly laughs a day to all my cancer patients and patients who want to prevent cancer. Belly laughter increases natural killer cells, our first line of defense against cancer. It also reduces stress and usually improves sleep, both powerful cancer fighters.

Although there's no question that environment and genes play a significant role in our vulnerability to cancer and other diseases, the emotional environment we create within our bodies can activate mechanisms of destruction or repair.[2]

It's true: our emotions work like medicines—good medicine or bad. And laughter really is the best medicine! Watching funny movies, going to comedy clubs where there is good clean humor, telling jokes, and simply enjoying life is the best prescription for stimulating the immune system. Comedians George Burns, Bob Hope, and Red Skelton were all a hundred years old when they passed away. Burns abused his body for much of those hundred years by smoking, drinking, and carousing. It may be because he had a joyful heart, though, that he was able to live so long!

TAKE COURAGE FOR TOMORROW

In addition to focusing on all the nutritional steps you can take to battle cancer, it's essential to maintain a hopeful heart. As you've seen, the war against cancer is by no means a hopeless endeavor. Stay curious about the things you can do to prevent it. Pursue those things; make those changes; remain joyful in the love of God. I have no doubt that if you do this, God's great promise will be true of you:

> Your wounds will quickly heal. Your godliness will lead you forward, and the glory of the LORD will protect you from behind.
>
> —ISAIAH 58:8

A **BIBLE CURE** Prayer for You

Father, You are the source of my health and the joy of my heart. The wisdom with which You made my body and the things on the earth that feed and strengthen it are beyond wonder. Science can only hope someday to discover all the miracles You worked into everyday foods and nutrients.

Not only that, but the fruit of Your Spirit are also the strength of my bones and the well-being of my body as well as my soul. To follow You is a blessing in every step.

Please give me wisdom not only in how to live in the fullness of health that is Your promise but also to expand that health, healing, and salvation to others around me. Thank You that I can be Your child and benefit from the wonders of Your creation.

I praise You, Father, in the name of Your Son, my divine Healer, Jesus Christ. Amen.

A **BIBLE CURE** Prescription

Your Soul Check

What are three passages of Scripture that have impacted your life as you read this book?

1. _____

2. _____

3. _____

Name three positive attitude characteristics that you want God to develop further in your life.

1. _____

2. _____

3. _____

What forms of exercise will you commit to pursue regularly from today forward?

1. _____

2. _____

3. _____

A Personal Note
FROM DON COLBERT

G OD DESIRES TO heal you of disease. His Word is full of promises that confirm His love for you and His desire to give you His abundant life. His desire includes more than physical health for you; He wants to make you whole in your mind and spirit as well as through a personal relationship with His Son, Jesus Christ.

If you haven't met my best friend, Jesus, I would like to take this opportunity to introduce Him to you. It is very simple. If you are ready to let Him come into your life and become your best friend, all you need to do is sincerely pray this prayer:

> *Lord Jesus, I want to know You as my Savior and Lord. I believe You are the Son of God and that You died for my sins. I also believe You were raised from the dead and now sit at the right hand of the Father praying for me. I ask You to forgive me for my sins and change my heart so that I can be Your child and live with You eternally. Thank You for Your peace. Help me to walk with You so that I can begin to know You as my best friend and my Lord. Amen.*

If you have prayed this prayer, you have just made the most important decision of your life. I rejoice with you in your decision and your new relationship with Jesus. Please contact my publisher at pray4me@strang.com so that we can send you some materials that will help you become established in your relationship with the Lord. We look forward to hearing from you.

APPENDIX A

Supplements below are listed in alphabetical order.

- Broccoli sprouts—OncoPLEX; available at www .drcolbert.com
- Cilantro tablets—available from Dr. Omura, www .micint.com
- Comprehensive multivitamin—Divine Health Multi-vitamin, Living Multivitamin; available at www .drcolbert.com
- Digestive enzymes—Divine Health Digestive Enzymes with HCL; available at www.drcolbert.com
- DIM—Breast Protect; available at www.drcolbert.com
- Fish oil (pharmaceutical grade, nonrancid)—Living Omega and Divine Health Pure (180 mg EPA/120 mg DHA); available at www.drcolbert.com
- Glutathione-boosting supplement—Max GXL; avail-able at www.max.com. Use distribution #231599.
- Green superfood—available at www.drcolbert.com
- IP6—available at www.drcolbert.com
- Kelley Protocol—contact Pam McDougal, nutritional consultant, at (208) 424-7600
- MAP—take five to seven tablets; available at www .drcolbert.com
- Melatonin, 3 mg—Divine Health Melatonin; available at www.drcolbert.com
- pH paper—available at www.drcolbert.com

- Plant protein—Life's Basic Protein; available at www
.drcolbert.com

- Resveratrol—Living Resveratrol; available at www
.drcolbert.com

- Vaxa Buffered pH—available at www.drcolbert.com

- Vitamin D_3, 2,000 IU—available at www.drcolbert
.com

- Whey protein—Enhanced Whey Protein, undenatured; available at www.drcolbert.com

APPENDIX B

Alkalizing Foods	
Vegetables	Alfalfa • Barley grass • Beets • Broccoli Cabbage • Carrots • Cauliflower • Celery Chlorella • Collard greens • Cucumber Eggplant • Garlic • Green beans • Green peas • Kale • Lettuce • Mushrooms Mustard greens • Nightshade veggies Onions • Peas • Peppers • Pumpkin Radishes • Rutabaga • Spinach, green Sprouts • Sweet potatoes • Tomatoes Watercress • Wild greens • Wheat grass
Fruits	Apple • Apricot • Avocado • Banana Berries • Blackberries • Blueberries Cantaloupe • Cherries, sour • Coconut, fresh Cranberries • Currants • Dates, dried Figs, dried • Grapes • Grapefruit Honeydew melon • Lemon • Lime Muskmelons • Nectarine • Orange • Peach Pear • Pineapple • Raisins • Raspberries Strawberries • Tangerine • Tomato Tropical fruits • Watermelon
Grains	Millet
Nuts	Almonds • Chestnuts
Sweeteners	Stevia
Spices and Seasonings	Chili pepper • Cinnamon • Curry • Ginger Herbs (all) • Mustard • Sea salt
Other	Alkaline antioxidant water • Apple cider vinegar • Duck eggs • Freshly squeezed fruit juice • Ghee (clarified butter) • Green juices Mineral water • Quail eggs • Soured dairy products • Veggie juices
Minerals	Calcium: pH 12 • Cesium: pH 14 Magnesium: pH 9 • Potassium: pH 14 Sodium: pH 14

Acidifying Foods	
Vegetables	Corn • Olives • Winter squash
Fruits	Pickled fruits • Cranberries
Grains, Grain Products	Barley • Bran, oat • Bran, wheat • Bread Corn • Cornstarch • Crackers, soda Flour, wheat • Flour, white • Macaroni Noodles • Rice (all) • Rice cakes • Rye Spaghetti • Spelt • Wheat germ • Wheat
Beans and Legumes	Black beans • Chick peas • Kidney beans Lima beans • Pinto beans • Soybeans White beans
Dairy	Butter • Cheese • Cheese, processed Ice cream • Ice milk
Nuts and Butters	Brazil nuts • Hazelnuts • Legumes Peanut butter • Peanuts • Pecans Pine nuts • Walnuts
Animal Protein	Bacon • Beef • Carp • Clams • Cod Corned beef • Fish • Haddock • Lamb Lobster • Mussels • Organ meats • Oyster Pike • Pork • Rabbit • Salmon • Sardines Sausage • Scallops • Shellfish • Shrimp Tuna • Turkey • Veal • Venison
Fats and Oils	Almond oil • Butter • Canola oil • Corn oil Safflower oil • Sesame oil • Sunflower oil All fried foods
Sweeteners	Corn syrup • Sugar
Other Foods	Catsup • Cocoa • Coffee • Mustard Pepper • Soft drinks • Vinegar
Drugs and Chemicals	Aspirin • Chemicals • Drugs, medicinal Drugs, psychedelic • Herbicides Pesticides • Tobacco

APPENDIX C

EARLY DETECTION THROUGH SCREENINGS

EARLY DETECTION IS extremely important. You need to know your family history and have regular checkups and cancer screening tests. The screening guidelines of the American Cancer Society (ACS) include:

- Yearly mammograms beginning at age forty

- Clinical breast exams (CBE) every three years for women age twenty to thirty-nine and every year for women forty and older

- Breast self-exams (BSE) beginning at age twenty

- Regular testing for colon cancer, such as colonoscopy and virtual colonoscopy, for men and women age fifty and older. (For a full list of tests, visit www.cancer.org.)

- Annual cervical cancer screenings after age twenty-one and Pap tests every two years. After thirty, Pap tests should be done every three years, plus the human papillomavirus (HPV) test.

- At age fifty, men should talk to their doctors about a PSA blood test with or without a rectal exam to detect prostate cancer. If you are at risk due to ethnicity or family history, do this at age forty-five.

Cancer marker screening is also available through American Metabolics. Their Web site is www.caprofile.net, or you can call 954.919.4814.

NOTES

Introduction—A New Bible Cure
With New Hope for Cancer

1. American Cancer Society, *Cancer Facts and Figures 2009* (Atlanta, GA: American Cancer Society Inc., 2009), 1–3.

2. National Cancer Institute, "Cancer Trends Progress Report—2009/2010 Update," April 15, 2010, http://progressreport.cancer.gov/highlights.asp (accessed June 2, 2010).

3. Richard Béliveau and Denis Gingras, *Foods to Fight Cancer* (New York: DK Publishing, 2007), 15.

Chapter 1—Squelching the Cell Rebellion

1. This quote can be found on many quotations pages on the Internet.

2. National Cancer Institute, "Quitting Smoking: Why to Quit and How to Get Help," August 17, 2007, http://www.cancer.gov.cancertopics/factsheet/tobacco/cessation (accessed June 18, 2010).

3. Béliveau and Gingras, *Foods to Fight Cancer*, 15.

4. Environmental Working Group, "Ethyl Benzene," http://www.ewg.org/bodyburden/cheminto.php?chemid+90001 (accessed May 20, 2006); Christian Nordqvist, "High Benzene Levels Found in Some Soft Drinks," *Medical News Today*, May 20, 2006, http://www.medicalnewstoday.com/healthnews.php?newsid=43763 (accessed August 2, 2006).

5. Agency for Toxic Substances and Disease Registry (ATSDR), "ToxFAQs for Tetrachloroethylene (PERC)," September 1997, http://www.atsdr.cdc.gov/facts18.html (accessed August 7, 2006).

6. Béliveau and Gingras, *Foods to Fight Cancer*, 15.

7. This quote can be found on many quotations pages on the Internet.

Chapter 2—The Cancer-Defeating Diet Plan

1. MedicalNewsToday.com, "Mediterranean-style Diet Reduces Cancer and Heart Disease Risk," June 26, 2003, http://www.medicalnewstoday.com/articles/3835.php (accessed June 2, 2010).

2. Antonia Trichopoulou, Pagona Lagiou, Hannah Kupeer, and Dimitrios Trichopoulos, "Cancer and the Mediterranean Dietary Traditions," *Cancer Epidemiology, Biomarkers & Prevention* 9 (September 2009): 869.

3. C. Caygill, A. Charlett, and M. Hill, "Fat, Fish, Fish Oil and Cancer," *British Journal of Cancer* 74, no. 1 (1996): 159–164.

4. Pollution in People, "PCBs and DDT: Banned but Still With Us," July 2006, http://www.pollutioninpeople.org/toxics/pcbs_ddt (accessed August 17, 2006).

5. Clara Felix, *All About Omega-3 Oils* (Garden City, NY: Avery Publishing, 1998), 32.

CHAPTER 3—DR. COLBERT'S TOP SIXTEEN
CANCER-FIGHTING AND -PREVENTING FOODS

1. Holly Wagner, "Black Raspberries Show Multiple Defenses in Thwarting Cancer," *Research News*, Ohio State, October 28, 2001, http://researchnews.osu.edu/archive/canberry.htm (accessed June 2, 2010).

2. Linda B. von Weymarn, Jamie A. Chun, and Paul F. Hollenberg, "Effects of Benzyl and Phenethyl Isothiocyanate on P450s 2A6 and 2A13: Potential for Chemoprevention in Smokers," *Carcinogenesis* 27, no. 4 (April 2006): 782–790.

3. Bettuzzi S. School of Medicine, University of Parma, Italy; Jay Brooks, chairman, hematology/oncology, Ochsner Clinic Foundation Hospital, New Orleans; April 19, 2005, presentation, American Association for Cancer Research, annual meeting, Anaheim, CA.

4. Thomas A. Gasiewicz, "Receptor-mediated Modulation of Gene Expression and Association with Biological and Toxic Responses," University of Rochester Medical School, August 20, 2009, http://www2.envmed.rochester.edu/envmed/ehsc/gasiewicz.html (accessed June 2, 2010).

5. I. Takahashi, M. Matsuzaka, T. Umeda, et al., "Differences in the Influence of Tobacco Smoking on Lung Cancer Between Japan and the USA: Possible explanations for the 'Smoking Paradox' in Japan," *Public Health* 123, no. 6 (June 2009): 459–460.

6. Katarina Augustsson, Dominique S. Michaud, Eric B. Rimm, et al., "A Prospective Study of Fish and Marine Fatty Acids and Prostate Cancer," *Cancer Epidemiology, Biomarkers & Prevention* 12 (January 2003): 64. Leonard Kaizer, Norman F. Boyd, Valentina Kriukov, and David Tritchler, "Fish Consumption and Breast Cancer Risk: An Ecological Study," *Nutrition and Cancer* 12, no. 1 (1989): 61–68.

7. Dagrun Engeset, Vegard Andersen, Anette Hjartaker, and Eiliv Lund, "Consumption of Fish and Risk of Colon Cancer in the Norwegian

Women and Cancer Study," *British Journal of Nutrition* 98, no. 3 (2007): 576–582.

8. M. A. Gates, A. F. Vitonis, S.S. Tworoger, et al., "Flavonoid Intake and Ovarian Cancer Risk in a Population-based Case-control Study," *International Journal of Cancer* 124, no. 9 (April 15, 2009): 1918–1925.

9. Johns Hopkins Medicine, "Cancer Protection Compound Abundant in Broccoli Sprouts," Johns Hopkins Medicine press release, September 15, 1997, http://www.hopkinsmedicine.org/press/1997/SEPT/970903.HTM (accessed June 2, 2010).

10. Gabriel Cousens, "A Healthy Perspective of Sprouts," as quoted in Ellen Schutt, "Proteins and Vitamins and Enzymes, Oh Sprouts!" *Nutraceuticals World*, May 2006, http://www.synergyproduction.com/pages/Sprouts-Article.pdf (accessed June 2, 2010).

11. Béliveau and Gingras, *Foods to Fight Cancer*, 102.

12. Ibid., 136.

13. S. E. McCann, P. Muti, D. Vito, S.B. Edge, M. Trevisan, and J. L. Freudenheim, "Dietary Lignan intakes and Risk of Pre- and Postmenopausal Breast Cancer," *International Journal of Cancer* 111, no. 3 (September 1, 2004): 440–443.

14. F. Boccardo, G. Lunardi, P. Guglielmini, et al., "Serum Enterolactone Levels and the Risk of Breast Cancer in Women with Palpable Cysts," *European Journal of Cancer* 40, no. 1 (January 2004): 84–89.

15. Milly Dawson, "Flaxseed: Protection Against Cancer, Heart Disease, and More," *Life Extension*, October 2008, http://www.lef.org/LEFCMS/aspx/printversionmagic.aspx?cmsID=116030 (accessed June 22, 2010).

16. Béliveau and Gingras, *Foods to Fight Cancer*, 141.

17. Adam Hayashi, Aric C. Gillen, and James R. Lott, "Effects of Daily Oral Administration of Quercetin Chalcone and Modified Citrus Pectin on Implanted Colon-25 Tumor Growth in Balb-c Mice," *Alternative Medicine Review* 5, no. 6 (2000): 546–552.

18. Béliveau and Gingras, *Foods to Fight Cancer*, 151.

19. Laurence N. Kolonel, Jean H. Hankin, Alice S. Whittemore, et al., "Vegetables, Fruits, Legumes and Prostate Cancer: A Multiethnic Case-Control Study," *Cancer Epidemiology, Biomarkers & Prevention* 9, no. 8 (August 1, 2000): 795–804.

20. A. H. Wu, R. G. Ziegler, P. L. Horn-Ross, et al., "Tofu and Risk of Breast Cancer in Asian-Americans," *Cancer Epidemiology, Biomarkers & Prevention* 5, no. 11 (November 1996): 901–906.

21. J. R. Zhou, L. Yu, Y. Zhong, et al., "Inhibition of Orthotopic Growth and Metastasis of Androgen-Sensitive Human Prostate Tumors in Mice by Bioactive Soybean Components," *The Prostate* 53, no. 2 (October 1, 2002): 143–153.

22. Institute for Responsible Technology, "Genetically Modified Soy Linked to Sterility, Infant Mortality," http://www.responsibletechnology .org/utility/showArticle/?objectID=4888#hair (accessed May 25, 2010).

CHAPTER 4—CANCER-FEEDING FOODS TO AVOID

1. This quote can be found on many quotations pages on the Internet.

2. ScienceDaily.com, "Does Sugar Feed Cancer?" August 18, 2009, http://www.sciencedaily.com/releases/2009/08/090817184539.htm (accessed June 22, 2010).

3. Roxanne Nelson, "Soft Drink Consumption Linked to Pancreatic Cancer," Medscape.com, February 10, 2010, http://www.medscape.com/ viewarticle/716806 (accessed June 2, 2010).

4. Cal Streeter and Michael Epitropoulos, "Detoxification in Relationship to Alkaline- and Acid-forming Foods," *Dynamic Chiropractic*, October 21, 2002, http://www.dynamicchiropractic.com/ mpacms/dc/article.php?id=15419 (accessed June 3, 2010).

5. Tullio Simoncini, *Cancer Is a Fungus* (n.p.: Edizioni, 2007).

CHAPTER 5—NUTRIENTS THAT GIVE YOU THAT EXTRA ADVANTAGE

1. Jean Anderson and Barbara Deskins, *The Nutrition Bible* (New York: William Morrow and Co., 1995), 319.

2. Edward Giovannucci, Meir J. Stampfer, Graham A. Colditz, et al., "Multivitamin Use, Folate and Colon Cancer in Women in the Nurses' Health Study," *Annals of Internal Medicine* 129, no. 7 (October 1, 1998): 517–524.

3. Alexis Black, "The Mineral Selenium Proves Itself as Powerful Anti-Cancer Medicine," NaturalNews.com, January 4, 2006, http://www .naturalnews.com/016446_selenium_nutrition.html (accessed June 22, 2010).

4. S. Y. Yu, B. L. Mao, P. Xiao, et al., "Intervention Trial With Selenium for the Prevention of Lung Cancer Among Tin Miners in Yunnan, China. A Pilot Study," *Biological Trace Element Research* 24, no. 2 (February 1990): 105–108.

5. MedicalNewsToday.com, "Vitamin D for Cancer Prevention," February 7, 2007, http://www.medicalnewstoday.com/articles/62413.php (accessed June 3, 2010).

6. Suzan Clarke, "In Tests, Vitamin D Shrinks Breast Cancer Cells," ABCNews.com, February 22, 2010, http://abcnews.go.com/print?id=9904415 (accessed June 22, 2010).

7. MedicalNewsToday.com, "Vitamin D for Cancer Prevention."

8. Eileen M. Lynch, "Melatonin and Cancer Treatment," *Life Extension*, January 2004, http://www.lef.org/magazine/mag2004/jan2004_report_melatonin_01.htm (accessed June 21, 2010).

9. Barbara L. Minton, "IP6 Is Highly Effective Alternative Treatment for Cancer," NaturalNews.com, April 1, 2009, http://www.naturalnews.com/025975_IP6_cancer_cells.html (accessed June 3, 2010).

CHAPTER 6—THE CANCER-BEATING LIFESTYLE

1. QuitSmokingStop.com, "Chemicals in Cigarettes," http://www.quit-smoking-stop.com/harmful-chemicals-in-cigarettes.html (accessed June 3, 2010).

2. American Cancer Society, "Alcohol and Cancer," http://www.cancer.org/downloads/PRO/alcohol.pdf (accessed May 31, 2010).

3. Zosia Chustecka, "AACR 2009: Diet, Nutrition, and Cancer—Don't Trust Any Single Study," *Medscape Today*, April 22, 2009, http://www.medscape.com/viewarticle/701722 (accessed June 3, 2010).

CHAPTER 7—TAKE A SOUL CHECK—AND A WALK

1. S. I. McMillen, *None of These Diseases* (Westwood, NJ: Revell, 1963), 7.

2. Bernie S. Siegel, *Peace, Love, and Healing* (New York: Harper and Row, 1989), 35.

Don Colbert, MD, was born in Tupelo, Mississippi. He attended Oral Roberts School of Medicine in Tulsa, Oklahoma, where he received a bachelor of science degree in biology in addition to his degree in medicine. Dr. Colbert completed his internship and residency with Florida Hospital in Orlando, Florida. He is board certified in family practice and anti-aging medicine and has received extensive training in nutritional medicine.

If you would like more
information about natural and
divine healing, or information about
Divine Health nutritional products,
you may contact Dr. Colbert at:

Don Colbert, MD

1908 Boothe Circle
Longwood, FL 32750
Telephone: 407-331-7007 (for ordering product only)

Dr. Colbert's Web site is
www.drcolbert.com.

Disclaimer: Dr. Colbert and the staff of Divine Health Wellness Center are prohibited from addressing a patient's medical condition by phone, facsimile, or e-mail. Please refer questions related to your medical condition to your own primary care physician.

Pick up these other great Bible Cure books by Don Colbert, MD: